PEACE
AND
POWER

CREATIVE LEADERSHIP FOR BUILDING COMMUNITY

SEVENTH EDITION

PEGGY L. CHINN, PhD, RN, FAAN

Professor Emerita
School of Nursing
University of Connecticut

JONES AND BARTLETT PUBLISHERS
Sudbury, Massachusetts
BOSTON   TORONTO   LONDON   SINGAPORE

Jones and Bartlett
  Publishers
World Headquarters
40 Tall Pine Drive
Sudbury, MA 01776
978-443-5000
info@jbpub.com
www.jbpub.com

Jones and Bartlett
  Publishers Canada
6339 Ormindale Way
Mississauga, Ontario L5V 1J2
Canada

Jones and Bartlett
  Publishers International
Barb House, Barb Mews
London W6 7PA
United Kingdom

Jones and Bartlett's books and products are available through most bookstores and online book-sellers. To contact Jones and Bartlett Publishers directly, call 800-832-0034, fax 978-443-8000, or visit our website www.jbpub.com.

Substantial discounts on bulk quantities of Jones and Bartlett's publications are available to cor-porations, professional associations, and other qualified organizations. For details and specific discount information, contact the special sales department of Jones and Bartlett via the above contact information or send an email to specialsales@jbpub.com.

Production Credits

Executive Editor: Kevin Sullivan
Acquisitions Editor: Emily Ekle
Associate Editor: Amy Sibley
Editorial Assistant: Patricia Donnelly
Production Editor: Karen Ferreira
Senior Marketing Manager: Katrina Gosek

Associate Marketing Manager: Rebecca Wasley
Cover Design: Kristin E. Ohlin
Composition: Shepherd, Inc.
Manufacturing Buyer: Amy Bacus
Printing and Binding: Malloy, Inc.
Cover Printing: Malloy, Inc.

Library of Congress Cataloging-in-Publication Data

Chinn, Peggy L.
  Peace and power : creative leadership for building community / Peggy L.
Chinn. — 7th ed.
    p. ; cm.
  Includes bibliographical references and index.
  ISBN 978-0-7637-5125-8
1. Feminism—United States.   2. Women and peace.   3. Community
organization.   I. Title.
  [DNLM: 1. Women's Rights—United States.   2. Decision Making—United
States.   3. Feminism—United States.   4. Group Processes—United
States. HQ 1426 C539p 2008]
  HQ1426.C48 2008
  305.420973—dc22

                                                                    2007015578

6048
Printed in the United States of America
11 10 09 08   10 9 8 7 6 5 4 3

Dedicated in loving memory to

Charlene Eldridge Wheeler
August 26, 1944 — March 30, 1993

Primary author of the first three editions of this book.

Her vision, wisdom, and persistent hard work were central to the conception and to the concrete reality of this book. Her spirit still lives within these pages, and within the hearts and minds of all who worked with her in groups.

CONTENTS

ACKNOWLEDGMENTS

This seventh edition has been possible because of the many women and men who, over the years, have inspired, assisted with, and diligently put into action the ideas of Peace and Power. First and foremost, Charlene Eldridge (Wheeler), primary author of the first three editions of the book, remains an inspiration and a dearly loved, although absent, companion in this work. Her words of wisdom and humor resonate throughout these pages to remind us of her deep influence on this work.

I owe a special debt of gratitude to the following people for their early encouragement and support, and for the special ways in which they shaped the fundamental ideas of Peace and Power during the years Charlene and I worked together: Wilma Scott Heide; Patricia Moccia; Lisa Albecht and the women of the Emma Collective; women of the Women's Studies Program and the Feminism and Nursing class at the State University of New York at Buffalo; various coalitions of women in the Buffalo community, including the Voices of Women Writers Coalition (1982) and International Women's Day Coalitions (1982–1986); Cassandra: Radical Feminist Nurses Network (1982–1989); the Friendship Collective (1987–1989); in Australia, Judy Lumby, Pat Hickson, and Cheryle Moss; in Denver, Carole Schroeder and her children Ben and Morgan; Fran Reeder; Marlaine Smith; and Jean Watson.

In the years since Charlene's death, there have been many special friends who have inspired the continued heart politics upon which this work is based: Elizabeth Berrey, Adrienne Roy, Chris Tanner, Janet Kemp, Sue Hagedorn, Richard Cowling, Kathy Maeve, Judith Claire (Australia), Lynne Giddings and Kate Prebble (New Zealand), Carol Polifroni, Adeline Rafael (Canada), Alicebelle Rubotsky, Mary Ann Anderson, Carrie Klima, Mickey Eliason, Carla Randall, Sue Dibble, Jeanne DeJoseph, and my beloved travel companions Sandy Talley, Nora Goicoechea, Shelly James and Kathleen McLane.

I owe a special debt of gratitude to the women who founded the ADYKE e-mail support list for older lesbians in the San Francisco Bay Area and to the group of ADYKE moderators to which I belong along with Mary Skinner, Duca Knezevic, Jane Tillis, Nancy S., and Karen Kane.

My family provides inspiration, love, and daily reminders that the work of Peace and Power is well worth the effort. To my partner Karen Kane, Allison Kane Larkin and David Larkin and their sons Cameron, Benjamin and Nathaniel, my son Kelleth, his wife Kheira and their daughters Sophie and Elodie, know that you have my deepest love and appreciation.

Peace and Power has come about because of vast networks of people who deserve special acknowledgment. Many whom I have not yet met in person communicate with me through e-mail or through others to share their experiences in using these processes. Many others I have met, but only briefly in a workshop or a class where I have discussed the ideas. Still others have worked more intensively in various contexts. A special word of appreciation is extended to all who have participated in classrooms, where for just a few weeks we experience what is possible when people come together to create communities of cooperation, inspiration, and support. To all who have contributed to this work, I extend my heartfelt appreciation.

PROLOGUE

Heart politics—the merging of power with openness, connectedness, and love—is part of the important work of evolving a way of creating and working with power. With this kind of power the criteria of success is the effect on living systems—human systems and the earth. Does our work and the way we exercise power promote life in all its dimensions? These are wonderful times to live in because there's real work that needs to be done: the work of learning how to live together and how to live in ways that allow the earth to survive.

Fran Peavey[1]

This book initially grew out of a desire shared by Charlene Eldridge (Wheeler) and myself to document, in writing, the women's wisdom that was passed on to us in the oral tradition and through lived example. For over a decade, until Charlene's death, we worked and played in groups of women dedicated to transformation. There was real work to be done, and they were wonderful times. Most of our work happened outside of formal institutions, in groups and collectives that formed out of the need and desire to see something happen— something that would not happen if we did not organize with other women to make it happen. Out of our experiences emerged the ideas recorded in these pages.

Wilma Scott Heide, a nurse and the third president of the National Organization for Women, became a dear friend who inspired Charlene and me to venture into self-publishing the first edition of Peace and Power. We founded Margaretdaughters, Inc.,[2] and sent Wilma one of the first printed copies of Peace and Power. She told us that when she first read the book, she wept, both from the joy of seeing feminist ideas presented in this way, and from the anguish of not having had the benefit of some of these insights in her early years of activist work. As we conveyed to her many times before her death in 1984, it is because of her own courageous living, and that of women like her, that we were able to do the work on which these ideas are built.

Throughout the years since that first edition, I have used Peace and Power processes in classrooms, committees, workshops, coalitions to produce major events in the community, cooperatives of women running a bookstore, professional organizations, as a framework for conducting research, and, most important, in my personal interactions with family and friends. I can say that, without exception, the processes have never failed to lead toward positive and constructive experiences. There have been many times when the shared hopes and dreams of those of us in these various groups did not fully materialize; but when we have tried to reach for the ideal, some aspect of the ideal has always emerged into reality. Most important, we have all learned a little something more about heart politics—about bringing together peace and power.

Over the past decade, virtual reality has blossomed and grown. The Internet, founded on principles of democratization, offers a powerful tool in achieving many of the ideals of Peace and Power—it provides for widespread distribution of information and knowledge (power), and communication of ideas, perspectives and possibilities originating all over the world. It brings up unique challenges for people interacting and communicating on a personal level.

For the past decade I have used the Internet and e-mail discussion groups to teach courses, conduct committee work and organizational business, distribute information and ideas, edit a journal, and participate in social support networks. In some of these online activities we bring Peace and Power to the center of what we do and how we relate. In others, we loosely use a few of the principles and processes. This edition contains major revisions that incorporate online interactions and address the potentials and challenges of working in virtual groups, based on my now-considerable experience.

There have been many circumstances in my work life for which I have not encouraged Peace and Power processes. These situations are so steeped in hierarchical traditions, with participants who are fully vested in maintaining the status quo, that it has been quite clear that my energies would be better directed elsewhere. Still, from time to time, there are small windows of opportunity in these contexts to call for value-based action, which, as an act of resistance, brings to light a glimmer of what might be possible. These situations always remind me of how the daily hum-drum of living in our times mimics entirely the larger, global picture, where the problems of the world seem so intractable, and so far from the value-based political realities that we seek.

When Charlene and I wrote the third edition of this book, the United States had entered into another war—the first Persian Gulf War. When the war "ended," peace did not exist, and still does not exist to this day. This is yet another grim reminder that peace is not merely the absence of war, and that redefinition of power is desperately needed. During that time, Charlene and I talked with many women who were also eager to explore how to create peace on earth by beginning within, where we live and work everyday, in ways that build on the values of Peace and Power.[3] We put many of the ideas together in the following list—a list that also forms images of communities for the future and that still inspires action in the very places where we live and work.

A Dozen and One Important Things You Can Do to Create Peace on Earth

1. Plant and nurture something that grows.
2. Practice the fine art of yielding—in your car, in conversation, etc.
3. Become active in a group that works on principles of cooperation, on principles of Peace and Power.
4. Fill your home, work, and commuting environments with visual and auditory images of peace and tranquility.
5. Do at least one thing to simplify your life and reduce your consumption of disposable products.
6. Do at least one thing to reduce your consumption of natural resources.
7. Move toward a vegetarian diet.
8. Learn and practice some form of meditation.
9. Learn and practice ways to reduce hostile interactions with others.
10. Exchange gentle forms of touch regularly.
11. Express appreciation to at least one individual or group every day.
12. Help three children learn three things on this list.
13. Pass this list along to someone else.

At the dawn of the year 2000, television stations around the world broadcast moving expressions from people all over the globe that, more than anything else in this next millennium, people yearn for peace. When we all learn to move beyond the celebration of a hoped-for dream to putting peace into action in everything we do and say, we will have peace on earth.

As this edition goes to press, the United States is again embroiled in war, this time more aggressive and more tragic than the last time. In preparing this edition, I have worked to express Peace and Power processes in the clearest and most direct language possible. The human project that this process embraces is the most important and urgent challenge before us all. It is my hope that this small book will inspire huge and lasting shifts in your work and life, so that yet another example will flourish in the world to show that indeed, real PEACE is possible. We begin here and now.

Notes

1. Fran Peavey, *By Life's Grace: Musings on the Essence of Social Change* (Philadelphia: New Society Publishers, 1994), p. 118.
2. Margaretdaughters, Inc. was created in 1984 by Charlene Eldridge Wheeler and Peggy L. Chinn. The name was a tribute to our mothers, Margaret Eldridge and Margaret Tatum, who taught us the importance of Doing What We Know. We published feminist writing and calendars and provided workshops on the use of Peace and Power until 1989, when we terminated our publishing venture and joined a large and respectable number of other small feminist presses that also succumbed to the realities of the publishing world.
3. Many people shared their thoughts about the creation of a do-able peace list, sometimes not aware that their conversation was influencing our thinking. We were particularly influenced by the words and wisdom of Connie Blair, Lorraine Guyette, and other doctoral students at the University of Colorado School of Nursing, Pat Hickson, Janet Quinn, Carole Schroeder and her children Ben and Morgan, Kelleth Chinn, and Christine Tanner.

CHAPTER 1

INTRODUCTION

Community. A word of many connotations—a word overused until its meanings are so diffuse as to be almost useless. Yet the images it evokes, the deep longings and memories it can stir, represent something that human beings have created and recreated since time immemorial, out of our profound need for connection among ourselves and with Mother Earth.

Helen Forsey[1]

If you have grown dissatisfied with the way things work in groups to which you belong and find yourself thinking there has got to be a better way, you are not alone. Many people are seeking alternative ways to build meaningful relationships and effective ways of working together in all sorts of communities and groups. This book gives you a "value map" to think about alternatives, specific guidelines for working with others to create meaningful community, and examples of real groups that serve as models of Peace and Power processes.

Peace and Power processes are specific actions that arise from carefully chosen values. In turn, the actions make the chosen values real—the values become visible and felt because people act on the basis of those values. These processes are designed specifically to overcome dynamics that set up advantage for some and disadvantage for others.

The practices of Peace and Power are both familiar and unfamiliar. They are uncommon in typical workgroups found in businesses, schools, and professional and community organizations, where the ways of interacting typically follow a model where a few leaders hold influence and power and most people follow what the leaders do and say. The practices in this book are familiar in places where people work on a more equal footing, which is often characteristic of places such as homes, where women conduct their own affairs.[2] Although the practices were developed from experiences of women, the processes of Peace and Power are specifically designed to overcome all types of imbalances of power in both private and public relationships.

The ideas in this book draw on the rich and varied feminist traditions that women activists and scholars have developed over many decades and in many countries. Many men have joined women in claiming these traditions, recognizing that the ways of interacting that are common in public life are all too often unsatisfying, damaging, and unhealthy. Feminist traditions value women's experiences and ideas and work toward a world in which women are no longer disadvantaged in any way. Feminist traditions value the full humanity of all people—women, children and men—and do not accept any condition that gives one group of people more privilege than others. The values upon which feminist traditions are built are those that assure fundamental human rights for all and that nurture full human potential, health, and well-being for all.

Women traditionally have been peacemakers, but women's peacemaking work and the skills it requires have been limited to home and family life.[3] Because this work has been invisible in public spheres, the skills required to be effective are not widely known or generally practiced in the world at large. But the values that are often found in places where women conduct their own affairs can be described. The skills and actions and abilities that go with those values are what constitute the Peace and Power processes described in this book. The close link between values and action is called "doing what we know, and knowing what we do."

Women in feminist traditions have been remembering and are continuing to re-member[4] the wisdom of doing what we know, and of knowing what we do. Although we may not always manage to do what we know, the wisdom survives and is being relearned with every attempt, with every reattempt. The knowing is so deeply buried under layers and layers of hierarchical learning and conditioning that the trying feels extremely tedious. It is at the same time exciting, affirming, and encouraging. It becomes easier with every attempt, especially within the context of a community that is loving and protective. Living and working in such a community is an experience that nurtures, that heals the mind, body, and spirit. Indeed, Peace and Power values and practices are closely related to the tradition of women as healers.[5]

Like much of women's wisdom, people have preserved Peace and Power processes primarily in oral tradition. The written word may endure in a concrete way, but it is static and vulnerable to destruction. For centuries, women scholars have recorded women's wisdom in written form, but much of that writing has not survived.[6]

The spoken word, on the other hand, while seeming to disappear once the words are spoken, endures within the heart and mind of listeners and speakers. The spoken word calls forth a response from the whole body. Once spoken, words cannot be destroyed unless every person who has heard those words is destroyed. Oral communication is also interactive, as the speaker and the listener attend to the responses of one another. The act of speaking is an emergence, a creation, and a form that gives rise to new acts, new thoughts, and new forms even as the speech occurs. The act of listening—hearing another's words expressed—facilitates a co-creation and allows a fine-tuning of ideas that combines each person's perceptions as words are shared. Speaking in groups, and even the language we use, is crucial to the co-creating processes of Peace and Power. You and others in your group will begin to create new words and new meanings for old words as you attempt to fully express values and practices that are grounded in Peace and Power. When listeners do not comprehend these new meanings, your actions and words of explanation help to make the new meanings clear. Fortunately, it is possible to convey the new meanings, because, in a sense, they are not new at all. They are part of everyone's experience, but have not had a language for expression. An example is the experience of peaceful, even energizing disagreement. There is no word for this in American English, but most people know the experience.

In this book, you will find old words with new meanings and new words created to more fully express meanings associated with Peace and Power processes. As a reader, you will not be able to observe actions that might enrich your comprehension. The stories included throughout the book will help to fill this void. This book also provides guidelines for thinking about and practicing new skills that are part of Peace and Power processes.

Although this book offers guidelines, suggestions, and practices that people have used successfully in many situations, it is neither comprehensive nor authoritative. Many groups have created practices to suit their own purposes. You might begin by using the practices described in this book and gradually create practices that are consistent with your chosen values and with your circumstances. Even the smallest shift in practice will dramatically influence how a group functions. As you begin to create processes in your own time and space, you will create meanings that emerge from your own wisdom and experience. You can use *Peace and Power* as a

handbook to inspire your own ways of living your values in work
groups, voluntary community action groups, and even at home.

As you and your group consider using Peace and Power, it will
be helpful for you to think about the following questions. These
questions provide a background from which you can clarify your
shared intentions to bring about fundamental change.[7]

Do we agree about our purpose?   It is common for members of a
   group to have different ideas about the group's purpose. Identifying a simple statement that reflects a common understanding
   of what you are all about is a good foundation for the work of
   Peace and Power. For example, suppose you are in a group that
   wants to volunteer to help distribute toys to children during a
   holiday season. Some people in the group might want to limit
   the group's purpose to a one-year project; others might want to
   establish an ongoing project that occurs every year. Getting this
   difference resolved early goes a long way toward preventing
   misunderstandings.

**Do we agree that we seek to equalize the balance of power
among everyone in the group?**   If people in the group can
   answer "yes" to this question, Peace and Power processes are
   for you—the processes are designed to do just this. This is easier said than done, and you will probably find that you will
   want to return to this fundamental value as a group over and
   over as you work out how to make it a reality.

How independent are we of external hierarchical structures?
   The more your group is influenced by a hierarchical structure
   (for example, a school, corporation, or business), the more difficult it will be to enact Peace and Power processes fully. Doing
   this will not be impossible, but realize that you may have to
   make major adjustments. Chapter 12 helps to address some of
   the challenges you will face. If you are relatively independent
   of an external hierarchical structure (for example, a community
   activist group, spiritual community, or intentional community),
   you will still be influenced by everyone's habits in hierarchical
   ways of being. But you will be relatively free to create your
   own processes consistent with Peace and Power and to challenge the traditions of hierarchy that individuals bring into the
   group.

Are we all committed to having time together?   It is not possible to develop a community unless you spend time together. For
   face-to-face groups, you may not be able to be together often,
   but you need to have some regular and agreed-on time to be
   together. Not everyone has to be present each time your group

meets, but everyone needs to know when and where the group meets. For online groups, everyone needs to be virtually present by signing on regularly and responding to the group as a whole.

Are members of the group willing to attend to the group's process? Peace and Power processes require taking time and turning attention to reflect on and discuss the group's process. You will be doing much more than just taking care of business. Peace and Power assumes that the group is striving to bring values and actions into accord with one another. This is only possible if you take the time to discuss what is happening in the process, and together carefully consider if indeed your values and your actions match. Example 1–1 illustrates what this means.

Do we seek meaningful change in ourselves and in the world at large? Peace and Power processes are designed to create practices that nurture and empower. These ideals may seem appealing and easy to embrace in principle. However, chances are that you and members of your group have lifelong experience with groups that interact in ways that alienate and divide, in ways that sustain privilege for some and disadvantage for others. In a group dealing with finances, as in Example 1–1, it is typical for those who are experienced, comfortable, and confident in dealing with finances to take charge and to claim considerable advantages for themselves because they are familiar with and in control of the group's finances. Those who are not comfortable and experienced with finances are often unaware of their disadvantage by remaining on the fringes where finances are concerned. Making a change to act and interact in cooperative ways that build strong community requires a commitment from everyone, challenges many practices that are habitual, and requires new learning for everyone. If you use this process, be aware that you, along with everyone in your group, will be called upon to make significant personal changes.

Example 1–1   Attending to the Group's Process

A group is nearing the end of a meeting in which the group discussed their finances. Discussion of money in any relationship can be difficult, and this was no exception. Rather than simply ending the meeting with everyone assuming that the business is done, the group takes time to have everyone reflect on what happened during the discussion that was positive, helpful, and consistent with the group's values, and what was not.

Continued

Example 1–1 *continued*

A couple of people comment about how thorough the finance chair's report was, and how well she explained it so that everyone could understand it. One person shares how difficult it is for her to think about taking a risk with money and shares her appreciation to the group for being patient as she works through her fears. Another person shares that he did not feel really patient because he does not have the same hesitancy, but he adds that he is working on being more understanding of others who do.

This discussion only takes a few minutes, but the group gains immense benefit because the discussion has helped them understand one another better, and they leave the meeting feeling good about their financial direction, and about the way they have worked together in dealing with their finances.

To Deepen Your Appreciation of the Ideas in This Chapter . . .

- Recall a group discussion that you remember as being very difficult, leaving everyone unhappy, perhaps angry. If you could replay your own participation in that discussion, what would you do differently? Why?
- Describe what "community" means to you—what would your ideal community be like? Do you belong to a group that might be open to considering the questions suggested above? What thoughts would you bring to the group in response to each of these questions?
- Think about the description of feminist traditions in the first part of this chapter. How does this description match, or not match, your ideas about feminism?
- Start a log of Peace and Power reflections. Write your questions, thoughts, feelings and ideas related to this chapter. As you go through each chapter, add to your log and review the chapters that came before.

Notes

1. This quote is from a collection edited by Helen Forsey entitled *Circles of Strength: Community Alternatives to Alienation* (Philadelphia: New Society Publishers, 1993), p. 1. This is an inspiring collection of

stories of intentional communities, activist communities, and religious or spiritual communities—all groups of people forming different ways of living and working together.

2. The links that I describe between Peace and Power processes and that which is feminist is informed by the work of Elizabeth Frazer and Nicola Lacey in *The Politics of Community: A Feminist Critique of the Liberal-Communitarian Debate* (Toronto: The University of Toronto Press, 1993).

3. See Elise Boulding, *Building a Global Civic Culture: Education for an Interdependent World* (New York: Teachers College, 1988). In her chapter entitled "Conflict, Diversity, and Species Identity," she addresses the two cultures of women and men and describes the work that women have done through women's culture to sustain society (pp. 62–64).

4. Mary Daly uses hyphens like this to convey a new possibility within a word, in this case meaning putting back together the pieces—the "members"— of what we know as women. Her books *Gyn/Ecology* and the *Wickedary* provide more enlightening study on her work with language and word usage. (See the Bibliography for references to Mary Daly's books.)

5. Diane Stein, *All Women Are Healers: A Comprehensive Guide to Natural Healing* (Freedom, CA: The Crossing Press, 1980). Although this book is primarily an exploration of the various paths to natural healing, Diane looks at women's roles and contributions to healing. She weaves rich historical evidence with well-informed speculation about the origins of healing as women's art. For a detailed history of women as healers, see Jeanne Achterberg's book, *Woman As Healer* (Boston: Shambhala Publications, 1991).

6. One of the most important books of this wave of feminism addressed the consistent and persistent erasure of women's knowledge and women's writing. In *Women of Ideas and What Men Have Done to Them* (Boston: Routledge & Kegan Paul, 1982), Dale Spender analyzes over three centuries of women's writing. She concludes: "We are women producing knowledge which is often different from that produced by men, in a society controlled by men. If they like what we produce they will appropriate it, if they can use what we produce (even against us) they will take it, if they do not want to know, they will lose it. But rarely, if ever, will they treat it as they treat their own" (p. 9). For several years after its initial publication, this book was out of print and very difficult to find. It was briefly re-released by Pandora Press in 1988. However, once again it is out of print—a grim reminder of the enduring reality of Dale's insights.

7. These questions were inspired by a discussion of group conditions that support consensus presented in *Building United Judgment: A Handbook for Consensus Decision-Making* by Michel Avery, Brian Auvine, Barbara Streibel, and Lonnie Weiss.

CHAPTER 2

PEACE

If I believe so much must change, I must be willing to change myself.

Francis Moore Lappé[1]

Copper Woman warned Hai Nai Yu that the world would change and times might come when Knowing would not be the same as Doing. And she told her that Trying would always be very important.

Anne Cameron[2]

. . . reflection and action, imagining and doing, are closely connected. We cannot act what we have not in some way thought.

Elise Boulding[3]

Peace is intent, process and outcome. The intention of Peace is the commitment to chosen values and actions that consistently bring about harmony, trust, and constructive solutions to differences and disagreements. The process of Peace is the interactions that flow from the commitment. The outcome of Peace is relationships that nurture ongoing harmony, trust, and constructive solutions to problems.

The kind of Peace that this book is about requires conscious awareness of what happens in a group, in a community. Peace requires that you know what you do as an individual when you interact with others. Peace requires that your chosen values guide your actions. Peace is the means and the end, the process and the product.

The acronym that follows defines the idea of Peace. Each letter of the word PEACE represents a commitment that guides the ways individuals can choose to relate to one another within the context of a group.

Praxis
Empowerment
Awareness
Cooperation
Evolvement

Praxis

Praxis is thoughtful reflection and action that occur in synchrony, in the direction of transforming the world.[4] Most people have limited understanding of praxis, because we live in a time when "knowing" and "doing" are rarely the same. In western cultures, the message "Do as I say, not as I do" is a familiar one. When you choose to convey the message that "I know what I do, and I do what I know," you begin to live your values. Praxis is values made visible through deliberate action. Your actions, chosen to reflect values of Peace and Power, become an ongoing cycle of constant renewal. As your actions are informed by your awareness of values, your thinking and your ideas are shaped and changed by your experiences with those actions.

As an example, suppose you become aware that you have been avoiding talking with and interacting with a person in your group who is new, who does not seem to be someone you would ordinarily get to know. You begin to reflect on what is keeping you at a distance from this person and come to terms with some stereotypes and prejudices that you want to overcome. As you begin to interact with the person, you realize that doing so is not easy; your old attitudes keep getting in the way. You continue to take every opportunity to interact, and as you do, you observe what you feel and how your actions are coming across. Gradually, you become more and more comfortable, and eventually are able to claim this person as a valued friend.

Empowerment

Empowerment is growth of personal strength, power, and ability to enact one's own will and love for self in the context of love and respect for others. Empowerment is not self-indulgence, but rather a form of strength that comes from real solidarity with and among those who seek PEACE. Empowerment grows not from an individual quest for personal strength and influence, but from active engagement with others whose values you share. Empowerment requires listening inwardly to your own senses as well as listening intently and actively to others, consciously taking in and forming strength. Empowerment is not power over other people, other creatures, or the earth. In fact, empowerment is only possible when individuals express respect and reverence for all other forms of life and ground the energy of the Self as one with others and with the earth.

For example, consider the process of ending slavery in the United States, and the end of apartheid in South Africa. People who were enslaved or disadvantaged had to act on their own behalf and claim their own personal power in order to be free. Some leaders in their governments and other allies were sympathetic to their plight and realized that the situation was wrong, and took bold actions to change laws and policies. Freedom for those enslaved and people of color certainly benefits those who were formerly oppressed and enslaved, but the fundamental benefit is the empowerment for all that can come from the social and political shift that assures human rights for all.

Awareness

Awareness is an active, growing knowledge of Self and others and the world in which you live. This means tuning in to the moment and valuing your own experience. This kind of awareness sees beyond the present to integrate the past and the future. This is a vital transformation in a society that treats the knowing and experience of minority and marginalized groups—and of women—as abnormal or nonexistent. With awareness comes a consciousness of double-speak, where what is defined as normal is really abnormal; where what is defined as peace is really war.

For example, there are immense social, cultural and structural barriers that make it hard or impossible for people with disabilities to do things in many communities. But as people with disabilities and their families begin to expose these barriers, others become more aware of the barriers and take action to make changes on behalf of people with disabilities.

Cooperation

Cooperation is an active commitment to group solidarity and group integrity. A group's commitment to cooperation grows out of mutually defined values, where each individual's viewpoint and abilities are honored equally. It means moving away from any action that exerts power over other individuals or groups. Rather, cooperation means encouraging everyone to use their abilities, ideas, and energy to join in creating a coordinated, cohesive whole. As individuals excel in a skill or ability, their achievements are celebrated by all and shared with others according to need and ability.[5]

As an example, people who want to combine their purchasing power and their preferences for certain foods and food sources might begin a community food cooperative. Each person participates in the work of identifying sources where they can obtain the foods they want, bringing food to a central location, distributing it to members, and keeping track of the financial matters involved. People share and rotate major responsibilities, but everyone takes turns doing the work that needs to be done. In this way, they benefit by reducing the cost of food and by having the kinds of foods they prefer from sources they know and trust.

Evolvement

Evolvement is a commitment to growth where change and transformation are conscious and deliberate. Evolvement can be likened to the cycles of the moon where new and old, life and death, and all phases are ultimately one. What remains constant is the cycle itself. As you experience group processes based on PEACE, you are changed. A group changes as circumstances shift, as individuals move in and out or become more or less involved, and as purposes or activities change. Growth and transformations are valued and celebrated with each new cycle. You create your realities as you live them. There can be no mistakes, no disasters—only opportunities for re-creation.

As an example, families evolve and change as the years go by. Some of the changes are welcome, others are not. But over time, the family remains identifiable as a family with a shared history and heritage. How families adjust as changes happen is important to the health and well-being of every individual in the family.

Peace Is Not . . .

PEACE, when you embrace Peace and Power processes, is very different from typical ways we have learned to "keep the peace." It is important to recognize and move away from the old ways that actually create dis-ease and distrust. Peace is not:

- letting things slide for the sake of friendship
- doing whatever is required to keep on good terms
- criticizing people behind their backs
- being silent at a meeting only to rant and rave afterward
- letting things drift if they do not affect you personally
- playing safe in order to avoid confrontation
- manipulating someone to avoid open conflict
- coercing someone to do what you want
- hearing distortions of truth without refuting them
- indulging another's behavior when the behavior is destructive
- withholding information to protect someone else

If you find yourself engaging in these old and destructive habits and you want to find new ways to create peace, this book is for you! Throughout the book you will find concrete ways to shift toward constructive, genuine peace-making actions.

Having Good Intentions Is Not Enough

Having the intent of PEACE is critical when you enter a group interaction. However, intent is not enough. Actions that flow from intent are essential; actions are the critical test of intent. Examine how fully your actions flow with your intent by asking questions like these:

- Do I know what I do, and do I do what I know? (Praxis)
- Am I expressing my own will in the context of love and respect for others? (Empowerment)
- Am I fully aware of others and myself, and do I bring these awarenesses to our discussions? (Awareness)
- Do I honor and encourage everyone's opinions, skills, and contributions? (Cooperation)
- Do I welcome practices that encourage growth and change for others, the group, and myself? (Evolvement)

To Deepen Your Appreciation of the Ideas in This Chapter . . .

- Think of a time when you had a troublesome argument or fight with someone you care about. Describe what your argument was about in a short sentence or two. Next, make two columns, one for you and the other for the person with whom you argued. List in each column the things that were most important to each of you (your personal values), and compare the two lists.

- Consider a situation in which you feel afraid to speak up and voice your opinion. What is it that keeps you afraid and unable to speak up? Where does your fear come from? What first steps might you take to be able to begin to speak up?

- Notice the ways in which your community makes it possible for people in wheelchairs to be fully engaged and active in your community, and ways in which your community maintains barriers for people in wheelchairs. Make notes about what you observe. To deepen your awareness of what someone in a wheelchair faces, talk with someone in a wheelchair to explore his or her own experiences of being engaged and active in your community. What does his or her experience teach you about your awareness, or lack of awareness, before your conversation? If you are not able to connect with someone in a wheelchair, consider the situation of someone with another kind of disability.

- Locate a cooperative group in your community such as a food co-op, housing cooperative (intentional community), or a child care cooperative. Explore what the group does and how the members work together.

- Continue your Peace and Power reflections for this chapter. Look back over your reflections for Chapter 1 and make notes of anything that has changed for you since you wrote those reflections.

Notes

1. Francis Moore Lappé, *Diet for a Small Planet: Tenth Anniversary Edition* (New York: Ballantine Books, 1990), p. 15.
2. Anne Cameron, *Daughters of Copper Woman* (Vancouver, BC: Press Gang Publishers, 1981), p. 53. Through the ancient myths of the native women of Vancouver Island, Anne Cameron offers "a shining vision of womanhood, of how the spiritual and social power of women—though relentlessly challenged—can Endure and Survive."

In her Preface, Cameron states: "From these few women, [the native women of Vancouver Island who told her the stories] with the help of a collective of women, to all other women, with love, and in Sisterhood, this leap of faith that the mistakes and abuse of the past need not continue. There is a better way of doing things. Some of us remember that better way" (p. 7).

3. Elise Boulding, *Building a Global Civic Culture: Education for an Interdependent World* (New York: Teachers College Press, 1988), p. 158.

4. Charlene Eldridge and I adapted this definition of praxis from *Pedagogy of the Oppressed* by Paulo Friere (New York: The Seabury Press, 1970), p. 36. Our adapted definition emphasizes the synchronicity of thought and action.

5. For a fun look at how to teach children and those who are children at heart the ways of cooperation, read *Everyone Wins! Cooperative Games and Activities,* by S. Luvmour and J. Luvmour (Philadelphia: New Society Publishers, 2007).

CHAPTER 3

POWER

This transition in our concept of power is radical. It involves seeing power not as a property we own, not as something we exert over others, but as a verb, a process we participate in. This is a huge evolutionary shift.

Joanna Rogers Macy[1]

The challenge for us in developing our personal power is our willingness to recognize that power is within us and in our courageous choice to forgive and release anything that prevents this power from fully manifesting.

Diane Mariechild[2]

Power in and of itself is neutral. We must take responsibility for our own actions and choose to know our own intent and the intent of any group before we simply follow a plan of action. Power-over demands that we do things we don't choose to do. Power-of-presence means we choose carefully and understand our intentions.

Grace R. Rowan[3]

Power is the energy from which action arises. The kind of power that energizes PEACE is different from power as it is used in the world at large. Power as it is used in the world at large reflects a hierarchical ideal. Defined in hierarchical cultures, power is the capacity to impose one's will on others, accompanied by a willingness to apply negative sanctions against those who oppose that will. This translates into a love of power, where the fact of having the power becomes more important, more critical, than what that power is used for or what results from the use of that power. Any measure that is necessary to retain that power is considered justifiable. People who are being manipulated or controlled often do not recognize these underlying dynamics because they are so thoroughly taught that the power structure, as it is set up, is the "only way." In this book, this type of power is called "power-over."[4]

The kind of power required to create and live PEACE comes from the power of love. What is valued is the capacity to be in harmony with others and with the earth, to join with others in directing your collective energies toward a future you seek together. In this book, this type of power is called "PEACE power."[5] PEACE power reflects a feminist ideal where the focus shifts to chosen values that guide the exercise of power, and to considering what happens to people's relationships when power is used.

This chapter will contrast these two types of power. These are not the only types of powers that might be imagined, but they are both very important to consider if your group is moving toward creating a balance of power in your relations with one another. Although PEACE powers are familiar, you may not be accustomed to thinking of them as power because of what you have experienced and learned in the traditions of the hierarchical power-over model. The PEACE powers are familiar because they are so central in the private world. They are not generally thought of as power because they are not yet the predominant modes of action in the private or public worlds. Even though PEACE powers may seem idealistic when you read about them, when they become visible through action, they create dramatic changes. They become very real.

PEACE powers and power-over powers are not opposites, but they do contrast sharply. When you focus on PEACE powers, you do not deny values that are associated with power-over powers that are also consistent with the values of PEACE. For example, consider the power-over "power of results" in light of the PEACE "power of process." It is often desirable and necessary to see results, or completion of a task or project.

Working with PEACE does not mean that you disregard the need to finish a task and see results. But you do not make the results or the completion of the task the center of your concern. Instead, how you and your group work together in completing the task is at the center of your concern, and you take the time and energy needed to assure that the work is done in a way that takes into account what happens with the people involved.

Power-over traits and practices are listed in the left-hand column. Features and practices of PEACE powers are in the column on the right, with a focus on the values and processes through which they are translated into action.[6]

Power-Over Powers	PEACE Powers
The **Power of Results** emphasizes programs, goals, or policies that achieve desired results. Achievement of the goals justifies the use of any means: "I don't care how you do it, just get the job done."	The **Power of Process** emphasizes a fresh perspective and freedom from rigid schedules. Goals, programs, and timetables are used as tools, but are less important than the process itself.
The **Power of Prescription** imposes change by authority; vested interests prescribe the outcome. The attitude is paternalistic: "Do as I say, because I know what is best for you."	The **Power of Letting Go** encourages change emerging out of awareness of collective integrity; leadership inspires a balance between the interests of each individual and the interests of the group as a whole.
The **Power of Division** emphasizes centralization, resulting in the hoarding of knowledge and skills by the privileged few: "What they don't know won't hurt them."	The **Power of the Whole** values the flow of new ideas, images, and energy from all, nurturing mutual help networks that are both intimate and expansive. Practices that nurture group solidarity are regular habits of the group.
The **Power of Force** invests power for or against others and is accomplished by a willingness to impose penalties and negative sanctions. One individual makes decisions on behalf of another individual or group of individuals: "Do it or else."	The **Power of Collectivity** values the personal power of each individual as integral to the well-being of the group. A group decision in which each individual has participated is viewed as more viable than a decision made by any one individual and stronger than a decision made by a majority.
The **Power of Hierarchy** requires a linear chain of command, where multiple layers of responsibilities are subdivided into separate and discrete areas of responsibility: "I don't make the decisions, I just work here." Or, "The buck stops here."	The **Power of Solidarity** shares the responsibility for decision making and for acting upon those decisions in a lateral network. This process values thoughtful deliberation and emphasizes the integration of variety within the group, while calling forth fundamental values embraced by the whole.
The **Power of Command** requires that leaders be aggressive and that followers be passive; leaders are assigned titles, status, and privilege (and higher pay!): "I will tell you what to do." And, "Tell me what to do."	The **Power of Sharing** encourages leadership to shift according to talent, interest, ability, or skill and emphasizes the passing along of knowledge and skills in order that all may develop individual talent.
The **Power of Opposites** polarizes issues. Individual preferences and insights are subsumed by the requirement to make choices "for or against." Language reflects the values of good versus bad, right versus wrong: "If you aren't with us, then you are against us."	The **Power of Integration** views all aspects of a situation in context. In the process of enacting self-volition, the individual integrates self-love with love for others and acts with respect for each individual's entitlement to self-volition.

Continued

Continued

Power-Over Powers

The **Power of Use** encourages the exploitation of resources and people as normal and acceptable: "If you don't want to work for what we are willing to pay, then quit. There are plenty of people standing in line wanting this job."

The **Power of Accumulation** views material goods, resources, and dollars as things to be used in one's own self-interest, as well as items to gain privilege over others: "I worked for it, I bought it, I own it—and I deserve it."

The **Power of Causality** relies on technology to conquer without regard for the consequences that might be carried over into the future. "Oh, the pill is causing you to retain fluid? Here, take another pill. This will make you lose fluid."

The **Power of Expediency** emphasizes the immediate reward or easiest solution. "Oh, radioactive waste? Let's just ship it somewhere else or dump it in the sea."

The **Power of Xenophobia** (the fear of strangers) rewards conformity and acquiescing to the values of those who hold the balance of power. "Be a team player. Don't make waves."

The **Power of Secrets** relies on the mystification of the process, agents, and chain of command. The agent who actually has the power rarely implements decisions or takes direct action, but assigns the dirty work to someone else: "I'm just doing what I was told."

The **Power of Rules** relies on policies and laws to dictate what must be done and to prescribe punishments for breaking the rules. A very few laws or rules are beneficial, but runaway rule-making creates absurd contradictions. "Do it because the law requires it."

The **Power of Fear** focuses on imaginary future disaster, and extreme actions are taken to prevent that which is feared and to control the behavior of others. "Let's bomb their cities: this will prevent terrorism."

PEACE Powers

The **Power of Nurturing** views life and experience as a resource to be cherished and respected. The earth and all creatures are viewed as precious, deserving of respect and protection, and integral to the well-being of all.

The **Power of Distribution** values material resources (including food, land, space, money) as items to use for the benefit of all, to share according to need. Material goods are valued as means, not as ends in and of themselves.

The **Power of Intuition** senses which actions to take based on the perceived totality of human experience. Although technology is considered to be a resource, it is not elected for its own sake or merely because it exists.

The **Power of Consciousness** considers long-range outcomes and ethical behaviors. Ethics and morality are derived from values that protect life, growth, and peace, and that are the basis for confronting destructive actions.

The **Power of Diversity** encourages creativity, values alternative views, and encourages flexibility. The expression of dissenting views is expected and encouraged. All points of view are integrated into decisions.

The **Power of Responsibility** focuses on demystification of processes and insists on naming and/or being the agent; open criticism and self-criticism are encouraged, motivated by love and protection for the individual and the group.

The **Power of Creativity** takes into account fundamental laws and rules that govern the society, but values actions and solutions created from ingenuity and imagination. Actions are created to fit each situation, with the knowledge that often there is a better way.

The **Power of Trust** focuses on building genuine human relationships where honest exchanges of thoughts and ideas are followed by consistent action. If trust is broken, then the relationship is renegotiated.

To Deepen Your Appreciation of the Ideas in This Chapter . . .

- Think of a person in your family or circle of friends whom you would call powerful. Which of the powers in this chapter does this person use? If possible, talk with this person about the things that they value most in their relationships with others in the group.
- Divide a page into two columns, one for power-over powers and one for PEACE powers. In each column make a note of how you feel when you are involved in each of the powers in this chapter. For example, for the power of rules, you might feel reassured by rules that are in place to keep law and order in your community, but also feel powerless against rules that are themselves unjust. For the power of creativity, you might feel overwhelmed trying to think of a creative solution to a problem, but also excited to imagine that some of your creative ideas might have some value for your community.
- Think about a group to which you belong. What is your role in the group? What are your intentions for how you act and interact in the group? Which of the powers tend to be practiced in your group?
- Continue your Peace and Power reflections for this chapter. Take some time to look back at your reflections from Chapters 1 and 2 and consider how your thoughts and feelings might have shifted.

Notes

1. Notes from an interview on "Womanpower" with Joanna Rogers Macy in *Woman of Power,* Spring 1984, p. 12. Joanna Rogers Macy is co-founder of Interhelp, an international organization that provides workshops on "Despair and Empowerment in the Nuclear Age." Bobbi Levi, who leads these workshops in Massachusetts, provided this interview for *Woman of Power.*
2. Notes from an interview on "Womanpower" with Diane Mariechild in *Woman of Power,* Spring 1984, p. 18. Diane Mariechild is a mother, teacher, healer, and author of *Motherwit: A Feminist Guide to Psychic Development* (Freedom, CA: The Crossing Press, 1981).
3. Grace Rowan, "Looking for a New Model of Power." *Woman of Power,* Spring 1984, p. 67. Rowan is described in this issue as "the co-founder of a shelter for battered women. She sees herself as a woman with power, and uses this power in her practice as a psychologist and for healing. She is a wise old woman on a journey to wholeness."

4. There are circumstances when exercising power over another person is clearly indicated, such as action taken to save a child from getting hurt, or to halt one person who clearly intends to harm another. However, power-over powers that are institutionalized as the only way, or the "good" way to relate to others, are seldom indicated or justified.

5. In this chapter, I continue to capitalize and cast in bold the letters of the word PEACE to emphasize this word as representing Praxis, Empowerment, Awareness, Cooperation, and Evolvement—the intentions and processes required to create community.

6. Charlene Eldridge and I first published a model of patriarchal power and feminist alternatives in *Cassandra: Radical Feminist Nurses News Journal,* May 1984, p. 10. This model is essentially the same model, but I have changed the labels to more clearly reflect what each tradition of power does, rather than using a label that is associated with the tradition from which it is thought to come. In initially developing these ideas, we used *The Aquarian Conspiracy: Personal and Social Transformation in the 1980s* by Marilyn Ferguson (Los Angeles: J. P. Tarcher, Inc., 1980) as a point of reference. Ferguson did not identify the prevailing power model as "patriarchal," but she did contrast the prevailing model with transforming power modes emerging in the latter part of the 20th century. We borrowed a few of her labels for various forms of power, but where we did so we conceptualized them from our own feminist frame of reference.

   When we were preparing the third edition of this book, Nancy Greenleaf provided the insights and suggestions that led to our inclusion of the patriarchal power of accumulation, and the feminist alternative power of distribution. In a letter dated February 7, 1989, after reviewing a near-final draft of the manuscript, Nancy wrote: "I found myself wanting to add to your power model . . . something that addresses the power of the 'free market'; a godlike 'invisible hand' that sorts the worthy from the undeserving and assumes 'self-interest' as a primary motivational force. This notion of power is inextricably combined with patriarchal notions, but it specifically addresses material (economic) well being. The feminist alternative is the power that accrues through material sharing of food, land, or space, and the de-emphasis on privatization of property. The feminist alternative would mean a commitment to bear witness to and expose material inequality."

   Charlene and I first named and described the feminist alternatives, now called the PEACE powers, from a wide range of feminist theory, as well as our own experiences working in feminist groups. See the bibliography at the end of this edition for a comprehensive list of the sources that influenced our early thinking, as well as more recent sources that have influenced the ongoing development of these ideas.

CHAPTER 4

MAKING THE COMMITMENT

Have you ever . . .

- been at a meeting where two people argued most of the time and nothing was accomplished?
- been at a meeting where you never heard what someone was trying to say because others kept interrupting her?
- voted against a motion that passed, knowing that your concerns were serious but were never heard or addressed?
- left a meeting thinking that you were the only one who was dissatisfied?
- left a meeting and then found out in the hall afterward what was really going on?
- left a meeting thinking "There has got to be a better way?"

There is a better way. The processes of Peace and Power are consciously formed ways of working that can overcome frustrations like the ones in the list above. Peace and Power points the way for you and your group to actively create, shift, and explore ways to put your values into action.

It all begins with individuals who consciously choose values consistent with the PEACE values of Praxis, Empowerment, Awareness, Cooperation, and Evolvement, and the values that are described in Chapter 3 as the PEACE powers. Creating a better way means taking personal responsibility for making these values visible through action. You can use the methods of Peace and Power without thinking about why, and the processes will create some improvement over groups that have used power-over methods in the past. However, the processes will become transformative for each individual and the group when you and your group make a firm commitment to consciously chosen values and to words and actions that are consistent with those values.

These processes are not a guarantee of totally satisfactory outcomes, nor are they automatic solutions to the dreadful meetings you may have experienced. In fact, the methods of Peace and Power, if used like a cookbook, will not bring about dramatic change. Also keep in mind that the methods of Peace and Power can be used in manipulative, coercive ways when they are not grounded in Peace and Power values. For example, if someone in a group says "I want to know your opinion," her underlying intention could be to know what she is up against in order to convince you of her way of thinking (power-over value), even though her words suggest she is interested in knowing what you think (PEACE power).

The problems that happen in groups do not necessarily arise from evil or malicious intent. More often, problems arise from values people have learned from imbalanced power-over relations. When power-over values are translated into action, what typically happens is alienation, advantage for some and disadvantage for others, and individual dissatisfaction.

Some groups work very well together, even though they use the typical ways of doing their work—following Robert's Rules of Order, electing officers in a hierarchical structure, and interacting in other ways that are linked to power-over values. Usually the effectiveness of these groups is due to the good will of the people involved or the fact that the people involved are very close-knit based on membership in a particular cultural tradition. But when problems arise, the traditional ways of addressing issues often lead to alienation and dissatisfaction, at least for some members of the group. Even more distressing, many people are left feeling at a loss to know how to better handle the situation.

Throughout the remainder of this book, you will see the ideal of creating a new reality through actions based on PEACE powers. The starting point is to be clear about the value or values you want your actions to reflect, and to begin practicing actions that reflect those values. Being clear about your values lays the foundation for addressing group problems in a way that builds community and unity.

The remainder of this chapter provides examples of specific actions and words that reflect values of Peace and Power. Some of these words and actions will seem familiar because they do occur in any group from time to time. What makes them part of Peace and Power is the values from which they originate.

Other words and actions in the examples will seem almost shocking. For example, it is very rare for a group to take time to discuss their process consistently—to reflect together on what happened in a discussion and how they might improve the way they work together. The common misconception is that there is simply not time to do this. To the contrary, when a group pays close attention to how they interact and links their ways of doing business with what they value most, their work becomes not only much more satisfying, but more productive.

In a group committed to Peace and Power, everyone understands their shared values, provides open disclosure of their intentions, and uses their words and actions in ways that genuinely connect to the group's shared values. As you read the examples in this chapter, focus on your own thoughts, feelings, experiences, and what you would like to bring into your life and into your group.

The Commitment to Peace and Power

A commitment to the Power of Process means:

Actions	Words
Giving yourself and everyone else in the group time to attend to a concern or issue that exists for any individual.	Chullie has a concern that I need to think about—I will call her during the week to clarify before our meeting next week.
Letting decisions emerge gradually, realizing that very few decisions are urgent.	I can wait to make this decision. How do others feel about waiting?
Inviting everyone in the group to express their ideas or concerns during the discussion.	Some people have not spoken about this issue yet. Do you have concerns that have not been heard by the group?
Acknowledging the things that happen that are consistent with the group's values.	Our discussion earlier about the grant application was so wonderful! Ann, your report was detailed and gave us all a clear understanding of what we are up against. Sidney, when we began to disagree, you stepped in to make sure that we all had a chance to speak to the issue, and helped us all understand one another by helping to clarify each point of view. And we all worked together to make this happen! Thank you to everyone!

A commitment to the Power of Letting Go means:

Actions	Words
Acknowledging but setting aside your own vested interests, in order for others in the group to express their interests fully.	I would like to protect personal time and not meet on Sunday. But I am open to knowing how others feel about this issue.
Supporting others who are new, or learning something new, in their work of taking on something you are already skilled at doing.	Michelle and I will be going over the bookkeeping system the hour before our next meeting. Would anyone else like to join us and begin to learn how to do this?
Expressing your misgivings or concerns about a situation in the group, but letting the sense of the group prevail when the group needs to move on to something else.	I have shared my concern about the expense of this project, but I sense that the group is moving toward doing this. I trust the wisdom of the group and seek support in letting go of my fear.

A commitment to the Power of the Whole means:

Actions	Words
Placing your own individual needs and interests within the context of the group.	I like to work alone and late at night. I could make posters, balance the accounts, or update the mailing list.
Seeking ways to do things together to equalize power within the group.	Nicole, how about updating the mailing list in your late night time? Making posters is a fun group project that we could do together. New members need to learn how to balance the accounts; could you write up some guidelines on this? Are there other ideas?

A commitment to the Power of Collectivity means:

Actions	Words
Taking into account the interests of every member of the group, including those who are not present.	We will consider this decision tentative until the other group in California has also discussed this issue and voiced their ideas.
Making sure that every concern is carefully integrated into every discussion and decision.	We have heard Jen's concern about the expenses, and her sense that the group wants to go ahead with the project anyway. I think we could go ahead with the project, but also make a clear plan as to what we will do if the expenses start to mount beyond what we can handle.

A commitment to the Power of Solidarity means:

Actions	Words
Addressing conflict openly and constructively, and, in so doing, working actively to strengthen the integrity of the group Keeping the group's principles of solidarity in conscious awareness as a basis for moving forward.	I am distressed because Janie and the publicity group have not explained their plan for this event. You always do a great job, but our not knowing your plan mystifies this important process and we have agreed to demystify what happens here. I would like you to report the plan at our next meeting so that we can all understand and help out where we can.
Celebrating shared values and joys.	I appreciate that the group did not ignore my concern about the expenses, and I feel good about supporting this project because of your response.

A commitment to the Power of Sharing means:

Actions	Words
Taking responsibility for leadership and tasks, including things you enjoy doing and can do well, as well as things you would rather not do but that need to be done.	I will take responsibility for the clean-up after the concert. I would like four people who have not done this before to work with me, because the requirements of the theater are important to learn. We need to maintain a positive relationship with them.
Encouraging others to join in passing skills and tasks along by assuming tasks from others	Randy, you have had responsibility for the inventory for two years now. I am willing to learn how to do this and begin to assume responsibility in that area this year.

A commitment to the Power of Integration means:

Actions	Words
Listening actively and deliberately to every concern or idea that others bring to the group, and taking active steps to understand and act on others' points of view.	Suzette, what I hear you saying is that you are losing faith in our ability to complete this project because we seem so scattered. Is this an accurate summary of your concern?
Taking actions that encourage bringing things together, rather than polarizing them into opposing points of view.	Since everyone can't be here at any time we have suggested for our regular meetings, how about if we alternate between morning meetings and evening meetings?

A commitment to the Power of Nurturing means:

Actions	Words
Treating others in ways that convey love and respect.	Pauli, I deeply admire the strength that you have shown in the face of this difficulty. Thank you.
Acknowledging that each individual's experience has uniquely qualified her to be where she is at the present.	June, I haven't faced the kinds of discrimination you have. It must tax your persistence and patience to keep trying to help us understand. Just know that when I seem resistant, I truly do want to know and understand.
Affirming and rejoicing in the knowledge that each person in the group has power to use, and power to choose how to use it.	Chris, I am sad to see you leave the group, but at the same time I am happy for your clarity in making such a difficult choice.
Using critical reflection (see Chapter 9) to bring forth the best for every individual and the group.	I am concerned about the quality of the presentation we are planning. We agree that our message needs to be clear and appealing, so I would like to discuss openly how we can improve what we have planned so far.

A commitment to the Power of Distribution means:

Actions	Words
Taking actions to overcome imbalances in personal material resources among group members.	Jan, Leslie, and I are able and willing to drive our cars and cover this expense so that all 12 of us can go to the retreat.
Using resources that are available to the group as a means, not an end.	Linda is willing to help us out of this tax mess at no charge. Rather than filing taxes for us, let's have her teach at least four of us to do what needs to be done.
Working to make resources that are available to the group accessible to all based on need, in the interest of the development of the group and each individual.	We have $200 in grant money to cover travel to do the interviews. How can we use the money to make sure that every-one who wants to participate can do so?

A commitment to the Power of Intuition means:

Actions	Words
Taking the time to think, feel, and experience the fullness of a situation.	I have been quiet for the past hour, reflecting on my growing sense that we need to go ahead with this. I am not sure why or how yet . . .
Taking actions that seem risky when your instinct tells you to go ahead.	I know this is a dangerous time to travel in that part of the world. I just feel that we need to participate in this project.

Paying attention to the intuition of others and taking their sense of things seriously.	Dallas, you are so clear about this even though the rest of us can't quite understand. I think we need to pay attention to your intuition about going ahead.

A commitment to the Power of Consciousness means:

Actions	Words
Talking about the values on which you are building your actions so that everyone can be fully aware of your intentions.	I am sharing with everyone all the details about how this works so that everyone can participate to the extent that you are willing and able.
Exploring with others awareness of feelings, situations, responses, and meanings in your experiences.	I am beginning to see a pattern in how we respond to folks who represent the funding agencies, and it makes me feel uncomfortable. I would like to put this on the agenda for our next meeting, and I will prepare some ideas and questions for discussion.

A commitment to the Power of Diversity means:

Actions	Words
Carefully considering another point of view when your immediate response is to reject it.	Wait a minute! I know I just said I don't agree, but maybe I am missing something here. Ann, tell us more about what you are thinking.
Taking deliberate actions to keep yourself and the group open to welcoming others who are different or new.	Before we move on, I want to back up because I think that new people are probably confused by what just happened. Would it help for us to explain more about what we just did?
Paying attention to subtle assumptions that may not hold true for everyone in the group.	I am becoming aware that we have assumed everyone has a partner to bring to the party. How can we make sure that people who are alone feel welcome and comfortable?

A commitment to the Power of Responsibility means:

Actions	Words
Keeping everyone in the group fully informed about anything in your personal life that might affect the group as a whole.	As many of you know, I am dealing with a difficult decision about my future, and I know this distracts me from time to time. Know that I welcome anyone bringing me back to the group if you notice that I seem to have mentally wandered away.

Continued

Actions	Words
Acting to make sure that nothing is mystified, that everything that concerns the group is equally accessible to every member.	The theater has strict policies to meet their safety standards. I have prepared a chart that shows everyone what their standards are, and the things we have to do to meet them.
Actively checking in and closing in a spirit of contributing to the growth and development of the group.	*Check-in:* I am Peggy. I have just left a difficult meeting at work, but am ready and eager for our discussion. I would like to make sure we discuss the poster design on the agenda tonight.
	Closing: I appreciate Monica's explanation of the theater requirements—that was very helpful to me in understanding why we have to do some of this stuff. Along the same line, I am still confused about the finances, and would like Ann and the finance group to give us more information about that next week. For my affirmation tonight—I believe in myself and our group.

A commitment to the Power of Creativity means:

Actions	Words
Imagining possibilities that have not yet been tried.	What does everyone think of this idea?
Drawing on everyone's ideas to craft new solutions to persistent problems.	Let's hear everyone's ideas, even the crazy ones, before we begin to make this decision.
Making better use of time, resources, and energy to accomplish what needs to be done.	Maybe if we all take a walk (stretch, dance, sing) we will feel energized to continue.

A commitment to the Power of Trust means:

Actions	Words
Letting everyone know your intentions and what you plan to do next.	I have to go now, but I will be back later today to finish what I need to do.
Keeping your promises.	I am back! I will finish this before supper.
Taking time to assure others of your commitment to your relationship.	I care about this group and being in it means so much to me. Even though it is hard to be here right now, I will stay and see this through.
Disclosing your underlying values when you speak or act.	Sue, I want to know your opinion. My opinion is different, but both of our opinions are equally valuable to the group as we decide what to do.

To Deepen Your Appreciation of the Ideas in this Chapter . . .

- Think of a time when you have heard someone say one of the phrases in the examples shown in this chapter. When this happened, what were the values of the person who used the word? Were the values consistent with the PEACE power shown here?

- Explore with your group ways you can all deepen your commitment to one of the PEACE powers that is particularly important to you. For example, if your group needs to focus on the Power of Trust, make a list of all the actions and words that would be important to the group. Be sure to focus on what you WANT to happen, not what you do not want. If your discussion begins to focus on what you do not want, shift to what you want instead.

- Highlight up to three of the PEACE powers that are the most important to you. Add to the examples in this chapter specific ways in which your actions and words can reflect those values.

- Continue your Peace and Power reflections for this chapter. Review your reflections from earlier chapters, and make notes of anything that has shifted for you since you first wrote the earlier reflections.

CHAPTER 5

FOUNDATIONS FOR BUILDING COMMUNITY

. . . . Imagine how it feels to always belong—belong in a diversified community, for it is the diversity in nature that gives the web of life its strength and cohesion. Imagine a time where everyone welcomes diversity in people because they know that is what gives community its richness, its strength, its cohesion. Imagine being able to relax into our connectedness into a web of mutually supportive relations with each other and with nature. . . . . Imagine a world where there was collective support in the overcoming of individual limitations, where mistakes weren't hidden but welcomed as opportunities to learn, where there was no reason to withhold information, where honesty was a given. Imagine a world where what is valued most is not power but nurturance, where the aim has changed from being in control to caring and being cared for, where the expression of love is commonplace. . . . . The very fact that you can imagine these things makes them real, makes them possible.

Margo Adair[1]

We can be sisters united by shared interests and beliefs, united in our appreciation for diversity, united in our struggle to end sexist oppression, united in political solidarity.

bell hooks[2]

Communities are defined by the values, concerns, or purposes that the individuals within them share. The phrase "global community" encompasses all who live on the planet earth and implies a general concern about the interactive global environment, economies, and politics. When groups of people within a community interact on more personal levels, the values, concerns, and purposes that bring them together are more explicit. Individuals begin to experience firsthand what it takes to reconcile their personal preferences and desires with the preferences and desires of others in the group.

Building communities for the future calls for everyone in the group to value both cohesiveness and diversity. Putting these values together into action brings forth solidarity. This means that you come together knowing that you will disagree, have different opinions, and see things differently from one another. Rather than seeking to agree, or pretending to agree, you acknowledge things that divide or that could divide you. You resolve to work together to understand one another and work toward mutual resolution of differences that get in the way, and you celebrate those differences that enrich everyone.

You also resolve to overcome fears, prejudices, stereotypes, resentments, and negative forms of competitiveness. Competitiveness that inspires fine performance and nurtures mutual respect and admiration for one another's accomplishments can be a strength within a group. However, when competitiveness nurtures jealousy, resentment, envy, rage, and hatred, the group is experiencing negative dynamics that are harmful. Through processes that overcome fears of differences, the group works to understand all points of view, to respect one another without coercion to change, and to find genuine common ground that sustains the group as a whole.

Common ground is formally expressed in principles of solidarity. Formal principles make your individual and group values explicit and help to guide the actions that flow from those values. Principles of solidarity provide a bridge between that which brings your group together and that which distinguishes each individual within the group.

Principles of solidarity provide:

- a grounding from which the group can focus their energies and resources,
- the ideals toward which the group builds,
- a guide around which to integrate all individual perspectives in forming decisions,
- a basis for giving one another criticism that is constructive and promotes growth, and
- a foundation for transforming conflict.

Principles of solidarity are statements of mutually shared beliefs and agreements that are formed early in the group's experience of using Peace and Power. Although writing them down is important, they are alive—they change and grow as the group changes and grows. Principles of solidarity provide an introduction and orientation to individuals who are considering becoming a part of the group.

New members may contribute valuable perspectives that can lead to shifts and changes in the principles, but the principles also form a grounding for stability within the group as membership changes.

The written document that contains the principles of solidarity is kept before the group; each member has a copy and works with it constantly. If your group has a Web site, you can post your document on the Web.[3] The document is particularly important as a source for building decisions (see Chapter 8), forming critical reflections (see Chapter 9), and when the group is addressing conflict (see Chapter 10). When each member's copy is almost not readable from the penciled-in changes that emerge over time, it is time to consider making a fresh copy!

Building Principles of Solidarity

Building principles of solidarity begins with everyone sharing ideas about the group, what interests them in being part of the group, and what they expect from the group. Each perspective is expressed as fully as possible. Then the group begins to identify those ideas around which there is common ground and those ideas that represent diversity from which to build common understandings.

Ideally, the group forms principles of solidarity in the first few gatherings. For an existing group that chooses to begin using Peace and Power processes, the decision to shift to this way of working together is the first step in forming principles of solidarity, and that decision becomes one of the principles.

The time invested to form new principles of solidarity or to reexamine existing principles of solidarity is the most valuable time spent in group work. Usually a task-oriented group that will meet regularly for a year or more requires two or three gatherings to form a beginning set of principles of solidarity and regular times set aside after that to reevaluate those principles.

Online groups have an advantage in forming principles of solidarity because of the ability to have every voice heard, to extend discussions of values beyond the limits of a face-to-face meeting, and to revisit principles at any time that the group's actions and values seem to be at odds. It is helpful to identify a convener (see Chapter 6) who is responsible for leading the discussion of principles of solidarity, because in an online group, several different discussions can be going on at the same time. A convener can watch to make sure the discussion of the principles of solidarity moves along. If the discussion gets stuck, or drags out for a long time, the convener can call for the group to reach a tentative conclusion.

A group needs to consider at least seven questions in forming principles of solidarity.[4] Each question becomes a section of the written document, but the specific principles will vary according to the needs and purposes of each group. In each of the following sections the examples of principles of solidarity are those of the Friendship Collective.[5]

Who Are We?

The name of a group implies a great deal about the group. You may need to define some words in your name to be clear about your identity. For example, the word "radical" in a group's name might be defined as "fundamental; going to the root." The definitions clarify who you are and who you want to be.

The group may also need to agree who the individuals within the group are or will be in the future. For example, a group formed to create and maintain a women's center in the community may deliberately seek participation from a broad base of women in the community, including women of color, women of all sexual identities, women of differing economic classes, and so on. A group that is working on the rights of lesbian mothers may actively seek the participation of non-lesbian mothers and also lesbians who are not mothers.

An important dimension of defining membership is clarifying how open the group is to integrating new members and when and how this will happen. A group formed to accomplish a specific, detailed, and long-term task may need to limit membership initially to a few people who are able and willing to remain dedicated to the accomplishment of the task. Although many groups will choose not to be closed, there may be times when the group needs stability in the membership, and the group might be open to new members only once or twice a year. Making a specific agreement about how long group membership will remain stable is helpful in preventing misunderstandings within the group and in communicating with others who are not group members.

The Friendship Collective was a group of 5 to 7 nurses who brought together skills of research and writing. We were a relatively closed group with relatively closed membership, since our work was focused on a specific task that involved research and writing. The group remained intact until the results of the research study were published.

What Are Our Purposes?

Defining who the group is provides a start in identifying the group's purposes. A women's center group may have the immediate purpose of finding a space, but then they need to identify the purposes for which that space will exist and how it will be used. If one purpose is to provide shelter for battered women, there are additional concerns to be addressed in relation to this purpose, such as whether to offer counseling or economic, legal, or educational services.

Consider your group's purposes in light of what is realistic. The members of a battered women's support group may want to see the group offer a full range of services to women and their children. However, the resources of the group may be such that the initial purpose needs to be limited to fundraising and educational work. Being clear at the outset about the limits of the group's purpose can help the group use their resources and energies in productive ways, rather than in working at cross purposes. The purpose of the Friendship Collective was to study the experience of female friendship among nurses and to publish the results of our investigation.

What Beliefs and Values Do We Share Around Our Purpose?

Values are fundamental to Peace and Power processes; stating your specific group values is important in helping each member of the group grow in understanding the meaning of these values. Having the beliefs and values stated provides a way for the group to examine how the values create changes in actions and group interactions.

The beliefs and values that formed principles of solidarity for the Friendship Collective were:

- We believe that friendships among women are fundamental to women's survival and growth.
- We value all forms of friendship between women.
- We value our own friendships among ourselves and are committed to living our friendship with deliberate awareness, examining and creating our experience as we go.

What Individual Circumstances or Personal Values
Do We Need to Consider as We Work Together?

Some values are not shared by everyone, but they affect the group and need to be acknowledged and respected by everyone. Different circumstances create different expectations and commitments. Different personal circumstances and experiences also influence what individuals need from a group to feel safe to speak, to act, and to *be*.

Some people may need careful limits on time and other personal resources. Women who have been verbally abused may need an agreement from group members that people will be careful about how loudly they speak and take care not to use sarcastic or assaultive voice tones. A person in a wheelchair not only needs space that is accessible, but also needs the group's awareness of the particular fears and challenges faced by someone in a wheelchair. A large person may not need specific physical arrangements, but needs the group's awareness of the discriminations she experiences and how the group can overcome these. Any person who is a minority within a group, whether based on race, age, gender, ethnicity, sexuality, social class, or education, needs recognition and valuing of these differences. Once the group has openly explored the range of personal circumstances of each person's life related to the group's work, then the group can agree on a common set of expectations that everyone values.

In the Friendship Collective the principles that grew out of personal circumstances and individual values were:

- We will not intentionally take any action individually or collectively that exploits any individual within the group or any other women, particularly exploitation that could arise from our roles as teachers or students.
- We will keep at a minimum any financial expenses needed from any individual in relation to our work and will openly negotiate these demands as they occur.
- We will be conscious of helping one another maintain a balance between the demands of our group work and our personal lives.
- We will maintain careful time limits for our gatherings that each member of the group mutually agrees upon at each gathering.

What Do We Expect of Every Member?

Time, energy, and commitment expectations can take many different forms. For example, group members might be expected to attend a monthly meeting and contribute to the work of a task group that meets for about three hours each week. For another group, members might be expected to attend a yearly meeting and work on one project during the year. Large groups that do not meet together but join in a network to promote communication might simply expect that every member contribute financially to the network, with the work of specific tasks done by smaller groups as they volunteer to assume a specific responsibility. Online groups might expect everyone to post check-in and closing messages every week, or whenever someone in the group calls for check-in or closing messages (see Chapters 6 and 9).

Bring to conscious awareness ways in which you expect each member to interact within the group. You have probably entered groups with an unspoken ideal or hope that everyone will be open and honest. In reality, most typical groups have hidden agendas and mystified processes. Making expectations clear is one step in the direction of nurturing openness and honesty.

Principles of solidarity that grew out of the Friendship Collective's expectations for interactions included the following:

- We will meet once a week until the initial stage of the project is planned. After that we will all meet face-to-face at least four times a year.
- We will take time to relax and play together.
- We are committed to using Peace and Power processes, including building value-based decisions and learning to provide constructive, growth-enhancing criticism for one another.
- We will address conflicts, feelings, and issues openly as soon as they reach our awareness, with the understanding that early awareness may not be perfect but deserves expression.
- We will share skills, leadership, and responsibility within the group according to ability and willingness, and will work to nurture these abilities in each of us so that we share them as fully as possible.
- We welcome any individual assuming specific tasks that need to be done that grow out of our mutually agreed direction, and support her initiative in doing so. We expect that each of us will keep every other member of the group fully informed as to the progress of her activities related to the group's work.

What Message Do We Wish to Convey to the World Outside Our Group?

Every group conveys a message to the rest of the world about who they are and what they are all about. Sometimes the message is accurate; other times it is not. A group using Peace and Power forms their message with careful and deliberate intent and constantly examines the ways in which they are conveying that message.

For example, a group that exists to develop services for battered women may decide to form a message that emphasizes women as physically strong, powerful, and resourceful. Another component of that message might be that women help other women, providing support and assistance in a variety of ways. These two messages become central in considering ways in which members of the group interact outside the group. These messages would grow out of the beliefs the group has about women in general, and also beliefs about women who are battered.

Principles of solidarity that the Friendship Collective formed in relation to their message included:

- We will work to form a message that is consistent with what we believe about female friendship and about feminist praxis.
- All public presentations will reflect our cooperative style of working, and will reflect our commitment to share skills, leadership, and responsibility.
- We will carefully and constructively criticize each public presentation or written document to examine the message we think we actually conveyed, and to re-form our own commitments and our presentation style as needed to more closely convey the message that we intend.

How Will We Protect the Integrity of Our Group?

Groups often encounter demands for time and attention from outside the group, particularly when their work creates social change. These demands may place unrealistic burdens on the group, and they may not always be consistent with the direction that the group wishes to take. Conscious awareness and anticipation of these possibilities help a group to develop agreements that can guide responses to outside demands. For example, a group that has been successful at fundraising might be asked to share their experience and knowledge with another new group in the community. If this happens once, it would not be a burden. But if it happens often, the group's energy could be drained responding to these requests.

Principles of solidarity formed by the Friendship Collective to protect group integrity were:

- All requests of our group will be discussed in a gathering with all of us present, and all decisions made regarding outside demands will be made by consensus of the group.
- Decisions about outside requests will be informed by a primary concern for the protection of each of us individually, our primary commitment to the work of our group, and our readiness to respond to the request.

- We will maintain our commitment to feminist praxis and to feminist methods in our work, and will carefully examine all situations that might result in an erosion of this commitment.
- We will seek external funding for our work, but will examine the demands placed on us in relation to accepting funding to assure that whatever demands these are, they do not compromise our primary principles.

Example 5–1   Online Process of Building Principles of Solidarity

A group of women started an e-mail list for women in the community who are getting ready to retire and who are retired for the purposes of creating social support and assistance. The list is moderated, meaning that all messages are reviewed by one of the founding women to make sure that all messages are consistent with the purpose of the list. When they start the list, they form a mission statement, and outline some of the values and concerns on which the list is founded.

For example, they are concerned about women's increasing isolation as they age and the risk for homelessness and poverty. They also realize that many women are afraid of using computers and will not join an e-mail list if they are made susceptible to spam, or if the list bombards their inbox with lots of messages. The group of moderators begins to refine their initial mission statement and gradually forms principles of solidarity that clearly state their concerns. The group also forms guidelines that they will use as they review and approve messages. At the end of the first year, the list has grown to over 800 women, and many face-to-face social activities have begun to form, providing women ways to make friends, find others with common interests, and obtain assistance meeting various kinds of needs.

The more the list grows, the more challenging the task of moderating messages becomes. The moderators realize that they have some different interpretations of some of their principles of solidarity, and there is growing confusion as to which messages to approve and which messages need to be declined or edited.

They start a private e-mail group to use for the purpose of clarifying these fundamental issues. One of the moderators

Continued

Example 5-1 *continued*

suggests that they focus on one guideline at a time, with each moderator posting a message paraphrasing the guideline and the related principles of solidarity so that they can all discuss the issues and clarify their different interpretations until they are all clear and have consistent understandings of the guidelines.

The group spends 3 to 7 days on each guideline, and within a month, they have refined the guidelines to everyone's satisfaction. During this process, there are about 5 to 15 moderator e-mail messages, requiring each moderator to spend about 20 to 30 minutes a day reading the messages and forming her response.

Regardless of the time involved, each moderator feels that what they have invested in this process is well worth it. They have renewed clarity and sense of unity. They realize that accomplishing this level of mutual understanding is vital to preserving their working relationship and to preventing unnecessary conflict in the future. They are confident they can all make decisions about approving messages that are consistent with one another. The new level of clarity will also make it possible to add new moderators in the future, orienting them with much more clarity about the procedures, as well as the reasoning behind all of the guidelines.

To Deepen Your Appreciation of the Ideas in This Chapter . . .

🙠 Focus your thinking on a group to which you belong that has not yet formed principles of solidarity. Can you identify answers to each of the questions in this chapter that characterize your group? Are the ideas consistent with Peace and Power values? What would need to change for the group to shift more fully toward Peace and Power?

🙠 What, for you, would be the most difficult challenges in forming Principles of Solidarity? Reflect on your personal circumstances and consider what you would need to integrate your particular needs into a group's principles of solidarity.

 If you are part of a group that is considering using Peace and Power, discuss together what each person sees as a personal challenge in doing so. Which of the questions for forming Principles of Solidarity are the most important for each person?

 Continue your Peace and Power reflections for this chapter. As you review your reflections from earlier chapters, what changes are you experiencing?

Notes

1. Margo Adair, *Working Inside Out: Tools for Change* (Berkeley: Wingbow Press, 1984), p. 284. This is a powerful, healing book that provides useful tools for bringing together the personal, spiritual, and political aspects of our lives, individually and collectively. Margo updated the book in 1993 to include her latest thinking on meditation throughout.
2. bell hooks, in her classic *Feminist Theory: From Margin to Center* (Boston: South End Press, 1984) discusses the experience and rhetoric surrounding the ideas of unity, support, sisterhood, and solidarity in the white women's movement, in her chapter entitled "Sisterhood: Political Solidarity Between Women." I have selected the term solidarity because of the connotation implied in the concept of solidarity: that we come together with our differences intact, respected, and integrated into a greater whole.
3. Group e-mail discussion lists are available at no charge through several providers on the Web. Most providers of group services include the e-mail distribution list, a home page with file storage capacity, simple database storage, group calendar, and many other features. See *www.topica.com, http://groups.yahoo.com* and *http://groups.google.com*
4. Kathleen MacPherson first identified four components around which the Menopause Collective formed their principles of solidarity. Her experience is related in her doctoral dissertation, completed in 1986 at Brandeis University, entitled "Feminist Praxis in the Making: The Menopause Collective." These Peace and Power components draw on Kathleen's ideas, as well as the ideas and experience of the Friendship Collective, who worked extensively to develop principles of solidarity.
5. For more information about the early work of the Friendship Collective, see "Just Between Friends: AJN Friendship Survey," *American Journal of Nursing* (November 1987, pp. 1456–1458) and "Friends on Friendship," *American Journal of Nursing* (August 1988, pp. 1094–1096).

CHAPTER 6

PROCESSES FOR GATHERINGS

In Peace and Power gatherings, you:

- give every perspective full voice.
- demystify all processes and structures.
- fully respect different points of view and integrate these into the whole.
- include attention to the process itself so that how you do things is just as important as what you do.
- rotate and share leadership according to ability and willingness.
- value learning new skills so that the opportunity to do so is accessible to all.
- share responsibility for the processes of the group equally among everyone present.

Meaningful communities value meaningful participation. This is often in the form of meetings where discussion focuses on issues facing the community and where decisions are made. Meetings and discussions also include meaningful social interactions that give people the opportunity to know and care about one another. Moving toward PEACE processes helps everyone understand Peace and Power ideals. You will see and experience values in action.

The description of Peace and Power processes in this and the next several chapters focuses on meetings and group discussions, but any of the specific approaches can also be used in informal interactions—in families, couples, social gatherings. Many people who have experienced Peace and Power in meetings take the ideas home with them, explain the reasons for shifting how they interact, and teach their friends, partners and children how to engage in Peace and Power ways. For example, a mother struggling with children who are frequently in conflict with one another can teach the children to use Peace and Power approaches to respect one another and to transform conflict. It is possible!

Peace and Power processes are also ideally suited for virtual, online interactions. The online environment facilitates many of the ideals of Peace and Power, particularly the ideal of having every voice heard. Since online interactions lack face-to-face non-verbal communication, virtual discussions rely heavily on words, and call for a deep commitment to being as clear as possible in forming messages using words.

When a group uses Peace and Power to its fullest extent, they do not have a structure of elected officers in the same way that many groups do. Instead, leaders emerge based on the needs of the group at any one time, and needs and leaders can shift at any time. For example, group meetings are led by a convener, and the responsibility to convene a meeting shifts in a rotation that is agreed upon by the group. The more that the group values everyone learning to be in charge of a meeting, the more often they will rotate convening to make sure that every member of the group gains this important skill. When a task requires specific knowledge, people in the group who have the knowledge or experience to do the task assume responsibility for it initially, but they gradually orient others to the task so that others can learn and assume the responsibility. For example, one or two members with experience in managing finances may perform financial management for the group initially, but they engage others with their work who do not yet know how to do this task, and gradually pass along this responsibility.

This chapter provides an overview of how face-to-face gatherings or online interactions can be conducted using Peace and Power processes. Chapters 7, 8, and 9 describe the major processes in more detail. Your group can form any number of ways to approach gatherings and online interactions, and can even use some of the traditional ways of conducting your business. The underlying concern is to work together in ways that express your values.

Overview

There are four basic components to the Peace and Power process. They are:

- check-in (described later in this chapter)
- rotating chair (Chapter 7)
- value-based decision-building (Chapter 8)
- closing (Chapter 9)

In addition, there are specific approaches to transforming conflict (Chapter 10) that build on these basic processes.

The processes described in this chapter are well-suited to groups of 6 to 40 participants (face-to-face or online). Smaller groups tend to work in less formal ways than those described here. Larger groups need to adapt these processes, using smaller break-out sessions for some parts of the meeting, combined with large-group discussions and reports from smaller groups.

Face-to-face groups sit in a circle so that everyone has eye contact. Usually one individual, the convener, prepares an agenda that provides structure for the group. This responsibility rotates among group members at regular times, such as every gathering or every month. The process for each gathering or online discussion has several distinct components that encourage each individual to put Peace and Power values into practice.

The convener opens a gathering or online discussion by beginning check-in, when each person becomes fully present in mind, body, and spirit. Check-in is a time for each individual to focus awareness on the purposes of the gathering, to share with the group any circumstances that might influence participation in the process, and to bring to the group intentions, expectations, or hopes for the time together.

Following check-in, the convener draws attention to the agenda and begins the process of rotating chair (see Chapter 7). In face-to-face gatherings, whoever is speaking is the chair. The primary purpose of rotating chair is to promote every viewpoint being heard, with each person's unique contribution being valued and necessary.

Group decisions are reached using value-based decision-building processes (see Chapter 8). Value-based decision-building focuses on reaching a conclusion that is consistent with the group's principles of solidarity and that takes into account all viewpoints and possibilities. Value-based decision-building focuses on what each individual and the group as a whole gains by the nature of the decision the group reaches.

The final component is closing, which is a deliberate process to end a gathering or online discussion and at the same time begin movement toward the next stage of the group's process (see Chapter 9). During closing, each person shares appreciation for something that has happened during the process of the gathering, critical reflection leading toward growth and change, and an affirmation that expresses a personal commitment for moving into the future.

The Convener

The one individual who comes to a gathering or who assumes leadership online with a specifically defined role is the convener. This role rotates so that each person in the group develops leadership skills. The convener's primary responsibilities are to prepare the agenda, to begin check-in, and, in some types of gatherings, to present a SOPHIA to focus discussion (described later in this chapter). During the gathering or online discussion, the convener assumes a leadership role, facilitating attention to the mutually agreed upon agenda. The convener actively attends to the discussion and calls for shifts in the process to facilitate staying focused on the group's purposes for this gathering. For example, when the convener notices that some people have not had an opportunity to speak in a face-to-face gathering, she might request a circling process (see Chapter 7) to give everyone a chance to speak. Or, when she senses that all viewpoints have been heard, she begins the process of value-based decision-building (see Chapter 8).

In face-to-face groups, the agenda can be written on a chalkboard or large sheet of paper (shelf liner or freezer wrap will do!) and posted before the time the gathering is scheduled to begin. The convener also identifies announcements or items that need to be mentioned without discussion and presents these just after check-in. In online groups, the convener posts the agenda in a message and calls for others to contribute to building the agenda.

Other members of the group can assume leadership roles at any time, but the convener remains particularly attentive to group movement. This does not mean that the convener behaves like the traditional "Chairman of the Bored"—calling time limits, reminding people to use rotating chair, or calling on people to speak. Once the discussion begins, the convener is free to participate in the discussion using the process of rotating chair (see Chapter 7), just as any other member of the group.

For groups that meet online, how you adapt the role of convener and the process for checking in depends on the kind of virtual structure you have (or do not have) for your interactions. An e-mail group list that is formed to accomplish a task can benefit from forming a structure that includes a time frame within which they want to complete their task, identifying the individuals who are responsible for different tasks necessary for completing the work, and an agreed-upon approach to discussing issues as they arise in the group.

The online convener might be anyone who takes the lead on a certain discussion topic, with several conveners going at the same time on different topics. If an issue comes up that is controversial or difficult, one or more members of the group can post a SOPHIA to help focus the group's attention on ideas and possibilities related to the issue.

The convener's unique responsibility is to make conscious choices to provide leadership for the group. Providing leadership that is focused on group process is illustrated in the following ways:

- Letting the group know when agreed-on time limits are near.
- Remaining conscious of requests made by individuals for shifts in the agenda, tasks, or processes, and making sure these are integrated.
- Helping the group to be aware of alternative possibilities throughout the discussion, such as minority viewpoints that have not received full attention, hearing from people who have not spoken to an issue, or choices that have not been considered by the group.
- Suggesting group processes that can move the group along, such as calling for "circling" or "sparking."
- Remaining attentive to possibilities for decision-building, and providing leadership for the group to do so.
- Shifting the focus of the discussion to closing so that the group devotes the time they agreed upon for this part of the process.

Conveners may use these guidelines in thinking about and planning for gatherings.

- Review notes from the last gathering or from recent online archives.

  ○ Are there items from other gatherings or in the archives that need to be addressed or items that the group decided to carry over for discussion?
  ○ Does the group need any new resources or information related to issues brought forward?
  ○ Has anything happened that will affect the decisions made in the past?

- Review group process.
  - What individual concerns or needs have people expressed that should be considered in planning for this gathering or time frame?
  - What group issues have people identified that need to be considered?
  - What strengths does the group possess that need to be sustained and supported?
- Plan the agenda.
  - What announcements need to be shared?
  - Are there special time considerations or individual needs to be taken into account?
  - What new items need to be introduced?
  - What specific tasks or responsibilities need to be completed before the gathering or before beginning the online discussion?

SOPHIA

In groups where discussion is a primary focus, a SOPHIA can be prepared by the convener in advance, and presented after check-in and after the group has agreed to the agenda. A SOPHIA is a 5- to 10-minute "essay" (about 500 to 700 written words) that comes from your own inner wisdom. Sophia is a Greek word for female wisdom; Sophia was wisdom in ancient western theologies.[1] In the context of discussion groups, a SOPHIA means:

Speak
Out,
Play
Havoc,
Imagine
Alternatives

A SOPHIA is intended to focus the group's attention on the topic of discussion. A SOPHIA is particularly useful in a class, a book discussion group, when a group is facing an important decision, or when a group is in a muddle about principles of solidarity. If the group has shared readings in advance of the discussion, the SOPHIA draws on those readings, but brings the perspective of the speaker to interpret possible meanings of the readings for individuals and the group. An important purpose of a SOPHIA is to raise questions for all to consider. The questions are also called subjectives (not traditional objectives). Subjectives are critical questions that arise from varying perspectives on the issue under consideration. There are no answers to subjectives; rather, there are many possible responses, all of which will be respectfully considered in the discussion. The SOPHIA, and the subjectives that it contains, offers to the group many possibilities to consider.

Checking In   *on-line*

Check-in is a brief (verbally 15 seconds or less) statement by each individual that centers the attention of the group on the shared purpose for being together. For online groups, each person's check-in message should be about 100 words or fewer. When you share your intentions for the gathering, everyone can integrate these into the whole of the gathering. Once this is done, there are no hidden agendas. At the end of check-in, everyone knows what needs to be on the agenda before the discussion starts, what the priorities are for the group and for individuals, and what the overall focus of the meeting needs to be.

Each person's check-in begins by calling (or typing) your name as a symbolic gesture of placing your Self into the circle, fully present in mind, body, and spirit. Then include at least one of the following:

- Share circumstances or events that are likely to influence your participation during the discussions.
- Reflect briefly on what you integrated or gained from the last gathering.
- Say what you want on the agenda, and what you are prepared to contribute to the discussion.

Check-in assures that everyone's concerns are considered fully by everyone in the group. In face-to-face groups, enough time needs to be provided so that each individual speaks, but each person speaks only for a brief time (about 3 to 15 seconds) so that everyone's presence is acknowledged before any discussion begins. Check-in is initiated by the convener and is an indication to all that the gathering has begun.

In online groups, check-in can happen at any time from anyone, but from time to time the group might want to have everyone check in so that the entire group knows who is really present for the group, and how each individual in the group is doing. In virtual groups, it is very easy to lurk. This may not be a problem for a group that is not focused on a task, but in a group that has a task or a specific focus, lurking is not helpful and plants seeds of distrust.

Checking in from time to time brings about a much better level of trust among everyone in the group and compensates for the difficulty of getting to know one another in a virtual environment. Checking in online can be more detailed than it is in a face-to-face group, because there are no time constraints online; a lengthy check-in will not prevent others from speaking. However, be aware that everyone in the group will have to read your check-in message, and if it is unduly long and tedious, your readers just might check out!

If you are joining an established group, check-in might feel intimidating. A lifetime of hierarchical group processes creates doubts about speaking openly in a group. Until you feel comfortable in a group you may only wish to share who you are and your purpose for being present.

One purpose for checking in is to address your own ability or limits in participating during the gathering. If you are not sure how fully present you are able to be, you might say, "I am distracted tonight, but I want to hear the discussion and participate as much as possible." You may choose to provide some details that will facilitate the group's understanding, such as, "My dog got out of the yard today and I have not found her. I do have friends searching, and it is important to me to be here and help plan the opening of the Center. I will leave at some point to call home and check on things, but I want to stay present as much as I can." Or online: "I will be moving to a new apartment over the next week, and may not be able to be online as regularly as I would like. I will drop in as much as I can to check messages, and will let the group know when I am online. I am very concerned to keep up with the information that the publicity group will be posting, so will make sure and check on that when I can be here. I will let you all know when I have everything set up to be back online regularly as well."

It is important to say something about what you hope for by being present. Knowing the circumstances that are influencing your ability to attend to the work of the group, and what you are working for on behalf of the group, the group can respond in a supportive and caring way.

Here is an example of how to share your reflections on a previous interaction to acknowledge what has happened, without imposing on others' time for checking in. Suppose that during closing at the end of the last discussion, comments were shared about Sally's constructive way of responding to another person. Sue reflected on the constructive approach that Sally used and practiced the approach at home. During check-in, Sue says: "I want everyone to know how helpful Sally's interaction with Mickey at our last meeting was for me this past week. My family was facing a similar dilemma, and I used Sally's approach to deal with the issue. It turned out great!" By Sue's sharing this experience of her own growth, the group can better appreciate the far-reaching influences of their collective actions.

Although every individual's check-in differs in extent and detail, it is vital for everyone to share their intention for each gathering. Silence or online absence during check-in leaves others wondering what you are thinking and leaves room for doubts about your intentions. Silence at this time interferes with creating solidarity within the group.

Responding to Check-In

Check-in does not occur in a vacuum. The group briefly focuses energy, time, and attention to what individuals share. When a person shares exciting good news, let your congratulations and shared joy erupt! When a person is preoccupied with some circumstance that may interfere with her participation ("My dog is lost"), the group may ask, "How can we best respond right now?" to find out what the person needs from the group. If someone shares a dramatic and important event—such as the death of a friend—the group may wish to suspend the agenda entirely or alter the agenda in some way in order to be fully responsive to the tragedy. Typically the group needs to take care not to let someone's check-in derail the meeting to a discussion that is not on the agenda. If discussion is needed based on someone's check-in, the convener (or any other member) can step in and note that this topic will be added to the agenda, so that everyone can check-in before any discussion begins.

Check-Out

There are at least two types of check-out. First, if you are not able to participate in an active way, it is wise to check out entirely, either from this discussion, or from the group altogether. Sleeping or reading a book during a gathering does not constitute being present or participating!

Another kind of check-out occurs when you are present and committed to the group, but you have specific limits on your time and energy for this particular gathering or for a time period online. If you will not be able to be online for a while, let the group know when you will be away and when you will return. If you come to a gathering and have to leave before closing, then explain your situation during check-in and give the timeframe to which you are committed. As the time nears, request the chair and share any closing comments. Give the group time to attend to your concerns or unfinished business or to make plans for finishing something in which you might be involved.

For example, a gathering has been scheduled to end at 10:00 p.m. Neva wants to leave the meeting at 9:00 p.m. because she is taking an exam the next morning and needs to get a good night of rest. Neva has been involved in planning for a concert that the group is sponsoring and wants to be present for that discussion. She shares her circumstance with the group and requests that the discussion about the concert be placed earlier than planned on the agenda so that she can be present for it. The group agrees to this priority and the gathering proceeds. As 9:00 p.m. draws near, Neva requests the chair and shares with the group that she is concerned that there are still some loose ends related to the concert. The group shifts attention to Neva's comments, wraps up the loose ends, and wishes her the best on her exam.

Example 6–1   Online Study Group

A group of students enrolled in a women's studies course decide to form an online study and discussion group. Since the class meets for 14 weeks, and there are 12 members of the study group, they decide to meet online starting the 3rd week of the class, and each group member agrees to be the convener for one of the weeks of the class. They all agree that the convener will send the group a SOPHIA no later than Monday night, and that everyone will contribute to the discussion throughout the week. They agree that everyone will check in sometime during the day on Monday. They also agree that everyone will show up online at least 3 times during the week.

The first week, Drew posts a SOPHIA that creates a wild flurry of responses and lively discussion that everyone enjoys. The same thing happens the second week when Sydney also posts a very interesting SOPHIA. At the end of that week, everyone realizes that they have lost sight of the "study" part of their group purpose.

Everyone agrees that they want to continue their lively discussions, but also focus on the questions and issues that they need to study. They agree that during check-in, everyone will post the study points they want the group to be sure and cover that week, and that the convener will organize all of the study points in the form of an agenda, with suggested time frames for each study point. After the fourth week, everyone is still enjoying their lively discussions, and also feeling that they are getting what they need to be well-prepared to complete the course requirements.

To Deepen Your Appreciation of the Ideas in This Chapter . . .

- How do you feel about speaking in a group? If you are very comfortable and tend to speak up readily, what could you do to encourage others to speak who do not feel comfortable speaking in a group? If you are very shy or afraid of speaking in a group, what would help you to be able to speak?
- If possible, find someone who feels differently than you do about speaking in groups, and discuss these questions together.
- How do you feel about using online messages and e-mail? If this is a challenge for you, what would help you to be able to participate more effectively online?
- Imagine that you are going to attend a meeting of a group later today or that today is the day everyone in your online group will be checking in. Write out what you would share during check-in. Make sure that you include all the components that are outlined in this chapter. Review what you would say. Have you included more detail than is necessary? Have you given enough information so that everyone in the group gains a better appreciation of you and your circumstances today? Do the intentions that you convey reflect how you honestly feel?
- If you were called upon to be a convener of a face-to-face meeting or an online discussion, what would your response be? If you feel experienced and capable of leading a meeting, what challenges would you face in shifting to a Peace and Power approach to convening? If you have little or no experience leading a meeting, what kinds of support would you need to be able to convene?

⤳ Continue your Peace and Power reflections for this chapter.
Look back over your reflections from earlier chapters. Are
you beginning to gain clarity about things that seemed con-
fusing earlier?

Note

1. Susan Cady, Marian Ronan, and Hal Taussig, *SOPHIA: The Future of
   Feminist Spirituality* (San Francisco: Harper and Row, 1986). Jane
   Caputi also elaborates on the ancient meanings of Sophia in *Gossips,
   Gorgons & Crones: The Fates of the Earth* (Santa Fe, NM: Bear &
   Company Publishing, 1993).

CHAPTER 7

ROTATING LEADERSHIP
AND RESPONSIBILITY

Rotating leadership and responsibility:

- assures that every perspective is given full consideration.
- equalizes and balances power within the group.
- assures the passing along of skills and knowledge to all who are willing and able.
- nurtures everyone's unique talents.
- challenges everyone to grow in their ability to participate, and to do things that they might not otherwise attempt.
- demystifies the processes of the group.
- provides practice and experience to meet challenges outside the group.

Rotating leadership happens in many ways, and is truly a process of "turning it over." Using practices that rotate leadership and responsibility reverses the familiar and long-accepted customs of hierarchical structures: a linear chain of command, wherein a single individual or an elite group manages the group and assumes leadership and control. Rotating leadership and responsibility turns over to each member of the group the rights and responsibilities for leadership, tasks, and decisions. It also opens the door for members to step back from leadership as needed, knowing that others in the group are able to assume this responsibility while they take some time off.

Processes of rotating leadership initially may seem awkward, cumbersome, and inefficient. The benefits are not always immediately obvious; they are benefits that emerge over time. For example, the benefit of having everyone acquire skills of leadership and critical reflection may only be clear when a conflict arises in the group. Once you experience processes of rotating leadership, and begin to experience the benefits in the context of a group with mutual intent and commitment to the values of Peace and Power processes, fears and reservations about the process gradually disappear. In fact, it becomes excruciating to try to endure the old ways when you have to go back and deal with the hierarchically organized world.

Rotating Chair Processes for Face-to-Face Discussion

There are several key features of a Peace and Power discussion.

- The agenda is built and affirmed during check-in.
- The convener facilitates announcements, focuses the discussion, and provides leadership for the process.
- Whoever is speaking is the "chair."
- Everyone in the group listens actively to the person speaking, and does not interrupt.
- The chair is passed to someone who indicates a desire to speak, has not spoken already, or has not spoken recently (not the first raised hand).

Following check-in, the convener focuses on any announcements. The group then reviews the agenda and identifies any items that need to be included that are not on the agenda, or reorders the agenda based on what people shared during check-in. If anyone has a brief item that simply consists of sharing information, this is a good time to mention that item. The group may set time limits and priorities on the agenda items.

In discussion groups, the convener then shares a SOPHIA (see Chapter 6). The subjectives (questions) at the end of a SOPHIA often spark discussion. In task-oriented groups, the convener focuses the group's attention on the first item of business. Then, in face-to-face groups, the chair rotates to whomever wishes to speak, and discussion begins. The chair continues to rotate to members of the group who wish to speak.

Once the discussion begins, you express your desire to speak by raising your hand. The person who is speaking is responsible for passing the chair to the next speaker. You pass the chair by calling the name of the person you are recognizing. If more than one person wants to speak, pass the chair to the person who has not spoken or who has not spoken recently—not the person who first raised a hand.

Passing the chair by calling a person's name is an important tool for a large group to help everyone learn everyone's name. In any sized group, it is a symbolic gesture that signifies honoring each individual's identity and respecting the presence of each person. Calling the next speaker's name is a clear signal that you have finished speaking, and that you are indeed passing the chair along.

You are not obligated to pass the chair to someone else until you have finished the ideas and thoughts you wish to share. At the same time, you have the responsibility to make way for all who are present to speak to each issue. Avoid making long, repetitive, or unrelated comments that prevent access to the chair for other people. If you tend to ramble and notice that others are not having time to speak, organize your thoughts and ideas in a journal and practice speaking more briefly in conversations outside the group. Then ask the group to give you specific feedback about how you are doing.

During the discussion, make notes of your own thoughts and ideas about what others are saying. Listen carefully to people who are speaking, allowing them time to complete their thoughts before you indicate your desire to speak. Frantically waving your hand in eagerness to share your thought is just as distracting and disrespectful as verbally interrupting.

At first, raising your hand can make you feel as if you have gone back to kindergarten. The benefits, however, soon become apparent. You can be confident that you will have a chance to speak, that you can complete your thoughts without interruption, and that someone with a louder voice will not intimidate you. Each person who wants to speak is assured of being able to do so. If you have a soft voice, you know that you don't have to shout to get attention. If you are unaccustomed to speaking in a group, you are assured of having encouragement and the time to practice those skills. If you speak slowly or often pause to gather your thoughts, you are assured that nobody is going to jump in and grab the attention of the group before you complete what you have to say.

Rotating Responsibility in Online Groups

Online groups have a distinct advantage in making it possible for everyone to express their thoughts and ideas. This can result in an overwhelming amount of e-mail or discussion board messages. Just as people vary in their comfort and ability to speak in a group, people have varying degrees of comfort and ability to communicate online. Some people send very brief, to-the-point messages; others prepare book chapters.

In an online group, every participant can compose messages that are short or long, with no limits. However, long and drawn-out messages in an online group are disruptive and annoying; they are difficult to wade through, and discourage others from focusing on other aspects of an online discussion. Group members may tolerate an occasional long message, but if you routinely post long complex messages, others will eventually barely scan what you have to say, or simply tune you out.

Online discussions also have the risk of overloading your inbox with scattered messages that wander through many avenues and sideline ideas. You can help avoid this for the whole group in several ways. As you read the messages that others in the group have posted, keep running notes to use when you form a response. Rather than responding to every message individually, you can form a single message that addresses several of your thoughts and ideas related to the discussion, and avoid repeating yourself, which can happen easily if you respond individually to every message. In your response, use people's names to identify a specific response to a message posted by that person.

Keep a notebook of your personal memos as you think about the discussion when you are offline. When you read something that is important to the discussion, make a note of it. Or, you might have an idea that you want to contribute to the group. Then compose a single message that summarizes ideas that have come to you over a period of a day or more.

Passing It Along: Notes and Minutes

Everyone who participates in a group, either face-to-face or online, takes personal notes. These notes facilitate the process of rotating chair. They are not a record of the discussion and are not generally shared with the group. They are used as a personal tool to remain in touch with thoughts you have while you are paying attention to what others have to say. Your notes make it possible for you to keep an idea in mind that you want to share without interrupting someone else who is speaking. They form a personal journal of your experiences in the group. They can also serve as a personal reminder of what it is you have agreed to do. These notes are a valuable resource during closing, making it possible for you to recall specific process issues to which you want to speak.

For example, suppose you are in a group discussion that focuses on a topic that makes you feel very uncomfortable. You are not sure how to share your feelings with the group at the time of the discussion, so you continue to listen (or read posted messages), and you jot down some of the feelings you are having and notes that anchor what is going on when these feelings come up. At some point during the discussion, possibly during closing, you decide to address your feelings with the group. You can look back at your notes to help you be clear in sharing your thoughts and feelings with the group.

For task-oriented groups, at least one individual can assume the responsibility for recording the proceedings of the gathering in the form of minutes. For gatherings that last longer than about an hour, passing this task along to different individuals in the group is helpful. Other kinds of groups may or may not decide to have group minutes.

Some groups keep detailed records of all ideas and comments, including who spoke and a summary of what was said. Other groups keep simple records of who was present at the gathering, the decisions made, and the major factors that contributed to each decision. The group's needs may even vary from one gathering to the next.

Minutes are not required, but you may want to keep them in face-to-face groups for several reasons.

- Minutes provide a permanent record for the group's archives.
- Minutes communicate information to those who are not present at the gathering, so they can be informed of what happened.
- Minutes provide a reference for the convener of the next gathering.
- Minutes help members figure out what they are supposed to do next.

In online groups, if you have a central archive on the Web of all of your discussions, you may not need minutes. If you also meet face-to-face from time to time, you can post minutes of the face-to-face meetings on your group Web site.

Task Groups: Getting Things Done

Sometimes the group (not any individual) rotates responsibilities to a committee, task group, or individual within the group. This is common when tasks require intense work and ongoing attention. The group determines what the task group is responsible for and provides guidelines that help that task group accomplish their work in concert with the group's principles of solidarity. The task group then decides and acts in accord with their responsibility. The task group brings back to the larger group an accounting of their work and issues that require a larger perspective.

Like face-to-face task-oriented groups, online groups that are formed to accomplish a task need to establish guidelines and time lines for their work. If your group uses an online e-mail distribution service that provides Web page capability (Topica, Yahoo, or Google for example), notes, minutes, membership lists, photos, and documents related to your work can be posted on the Web site. This level of accessibility to information is wonderful for groups using Peace and Power; it ties in to the powers of sharing, distribution, nurturing, and many others.

One benefit of having task groups for specific or ongoing work is the passing along of skills. A task group usually gets involved in doing intensive work that requires special skills and knowledge. Learning a skill is done by participating in the work, not by simply hearing about the results of the work. Hearing or reading a finance task group's report, no matter how detailed, does not help anyone learn how to balance the books!

Task groups that are most effective in getting the job done and in passing along skills are those that have a balance of people who are experienced at the task and those who are learning. This requires a gradual shift over time in who is involved with any task group so that the work and responsibility rotate.

Active Listening

Active listening is a vital part of the process of rotating responsibility. In a face-to-face group, active listening means being fully tuned in to a speaker and verbally checking out your perception of what you heard. It requires deliberate awareness of how you perceive what other people say. When you are ready to confirm what you heard, request the chair and paraphrase in your own words what you understood. The speaker can affirm your perception or clarify any misunderstanding. Other people in the group can also contribute to helping everyone get clear about the intended message.

In online interactions, use the same practice of confirming what you read in someone's message. Share in your own words what you understand, and ask others in the group to help clarify.

The Tyrannies of Silence and Repetition

Working effectively together is difficult, if not impossible, if some people in the group consistently do not speak to issues. When you do not express your viewpoint, your silence deprives the group of the benefit of your ideas. Silence, or online absence, also leaves people wondering what you are really thinking, or even worse, making assumptions about your thoughts and opinions.

Remember: this process does not function on the notions of majority and minority. Even if you are the only one who holds an opinion, the group must take your ideas and thoughts seriously. The group considers every viewpoint, regardless of how many or how few hold that viewpoint. Even more important, Peace and Power processes are based on valuing each individual, and others can only know what you uniquely offer to the group when you share your opinions, thoughts, and ideas.

At the same time, it is not necessary for every individual to address every issue. If someone has already expressed your viewpoint, you need not repeat what someone else has already said, although it is often important that you indicate to the group that you agree with that person. If you agree but have a different thought or concern to add, you need to speak to have your additional thought considered in the discussion.

Shifting to "Every-Logue"

When two people are together, dialogue is highly desirable. It is important for each person to contribute to the discussion; otherwise, it is not a discussion. In a group larger than two, the same principle holds: everyone needs to contribute to the discussion. Otherwise, it is not a discussion. In a group of more than two people, dialogue is like a monologue in a twosome—one or two people dominate the discussion so that other voices are not heard. Any form of domination in a group discussion models power-over tactics of traditional meetings. Monologue or dialogue in a group alienates other participants, promotes argument and debate between and among individuals, and prevents other viewpoints from being heard. Rotating chair is designed to facilitate "every-logue," assuring that every person speaks, with a sufficient balance of attention devoted to every point of view.

When two people become engaged in energetic opposition to one another's ideas (face-to-face or online), it is time for other voices to come forward. Conflict can be growthful and desirable (see Chapter 10), but when two individuals in conflict get caught up in the conflict itself, others in the group cannot easily participate in the discussion. As other people speak, the group can define what the issue really is. Also, the two people who are in conflict have an opportunity to reflect on their own positions, consider the thoughts and feelings of other group members, and decide if their thoughts and feelings are helping or hindering group process.

When you notice that two people are engaging in dialogue to the exclusion of others, request the chair or post a message. Share your observation of what is happening and convey your perspective on the issue. Then invite others to speak as well. Almost always, when other people speak, everyone gains insight and clarity about the issue, and many creative possibilities begin to emerge.

Sometimes one or two individuals have specific information about a certain issue. Directing a question to an individual and engaging in information exchange is different from exclusive dialogue. Information exchange is simply that—information exchange. The pitfall to watch for is when a group consistently defers to one or two individuals as the "knowledgeable ones." This is a signal that sharing of information and skills is not happening, and the group needs to give attention to providing the opportunity for everyone to share points of view or information.

Variations

Rotating leadership and responsibility can be done in many different ways, and you will create ways not included here. The idea is to find ways that are effective in expressing the values and intents of Peace and Power (see the value-based actions at the beginning of Chapter 6). Variations are often needed when the group is small (fewer than 6), or large (more than about 40). Small groups tend to be less formal, and often rely on "dinner-table" styles of discussion. When this happens, everyone gets to speak, but the discussion may wander. In large groups, some people may not have the opportunity to speak, and shy people may find it very difficult to speak. Here are some methods for promoting discussion that are consistent with Peace and Power processes.

Sparking

In face-to-face groups, when an issue or a topic generates a great deal of excitement in the group, the discussion often moves naturally into a style that reflects the high energy of excitement. Many individuals begin to speak, sometimes at once, often spouting words and ideas into the air like a fountain. In an online group, you suddenly see a surge of message posts on the same topic.

This type of discussion is referred to as sparking. When it begins to happen naturally, it should be allowed to continue as long as the discussion is giving the group new ideas and energy to move forward. When some individuals begin to lose interest, however, or the ideas are beginning to be repetitive, it is time for the convener or another group member to assume leadership, asking the group to cease sparking and return to the more focused style of rotating chair or online discussion.

You can bring an idea or topic to the group that needs sparking. Ask the group to enter this style of discussion for a specific time, or plan to include sparking around the idea in the future.

Sparking is a valuable process for creating ideas and energy, but it does not work well to help everyone participate equally or to be heard. When you use it, do so with deliberate intent, and make sure everyone in the group is aware that this is what is going on. When it is time to cease, you can use circling to transition back to rotating chair and less intense discussion.

Circling

Circling in a face-to-face group is what happens when the group suspends discussion and rotation of the chair, inviting everyone in the group to take a turn in speaking to an issue. People listen to one another in turn. Nobody responds to or discusses any comment or idea until everyone has spoken. If you have questions or want clarification, make a note to yourself so you can seek clarification after everyone has spoken. Although it is usually the convener, any group member who perceives that the group needs to focus and clarify may request the group to circle. Whoever calls for a circle then shares an idea of what the focus of the circle needs to be.

The process of circling is easily accomplished online. When someone in the group asks everyone in the group to speak to an issue or an idea, it is very important not to simply lurk and remain electronically silent. Your virtual presence in an online group is as important as your presence in a face-to-face group, perhaps even more so. The level of trust that an online group develops depends on everyone showing up online. You are known by the contributions you make to the online processes, and it is your responsibility to convey to others in the group what you are thinking and feeling, and to interact with the group process in ways that express your intentions with the group.

During circling, everyone speaks or writes very briefly, with comments limited to the focus for which circling has been requested. This provides a connection with all of the points of view at that particular time. It also provides time for individuals to clarify their ideas in their own minds before speaking. Even if you have nothing specific to contribute at this time, it is important for you to contribute during circling. You might simply say: "I am not clear about this issue and need more time."

When the discussion seems to be nearing time to consider building a decision, but this is not yet clear, someone can request a circle to simply find out if people feel ready to move toward closure on the issue. At the end of sparking, circling can be a time for everyone to share which of the ideas expressed "sparked" the most.

Circling is especially helpful when tensions are running high, with two or three individuals at the center of the struggle. You can use circling to interrupt exclusive dialogue that often begins during times of tension. Circling gives every individual in the group the responsibility and the opportunity to speak, to share insights of the moment, or to express feelings that may not already be apparent. Circling provides the opportunity for people at the center of a struggle to pay close attention to what others have to offer, and time to do some inner work with respect to the struggle.

Time Signal

Despite the best of intentions, individuals sometimes do get carried away. In face-to-face groups, if a group is having difficulty with extended minispeeches that interfere with everyone having the opportunity to speak, they can agree to use a time signal to help speakers remember to bring their comments to a close so that others can speak. A time signal is a simple "T" formed with the hands.

In online groups, messages that contain book chapters consume everyone else's reading time. The group can agree on a virtual time signal to remind everyone to keep their posts within reason.

A conscious decision to use a time signal avoids the slip into unconscious patterns of interacting in face-to-face groups. Out-shouting, long tirades, or other verbal forms of domination are common power-over habits that many well-intentioned people have cultivated. When a group is using rotating chair, a common unconscious habit used to try to interrupt long-winded speakers is hand-waving to ask for the chair while the speaker is still speaking. Not only is hand-waving disrespectful of the speaker, it is disruptive to the process and to the group, and places the responsibility for monitoring another speaker on those who are eager to speak.

When a group recognizes that long-winded speeches or excessively long posts are interfering with their process, then a consciously chosen signal is a respectful way to begin to shift patterns of response to others in the group. The time signal does interrupt the speaker, but it has several features that are different from the power-over verbal interruptions or distracting hand-waving. It is a signal that is preferably agreed on by the group because they share a desire to equalize access to discussion. The signal itself is quiet: It does not unnecessarily escalate emotions in the group with loud sound or frantic movement. Importantly, it is a signal that simply reminds the speaker of an agreed-on responsibility to respect others in the group and give way for others to speak.

The person who gives the time signal is not trying to overtake the speaker by asking to speak. The time signal is not a request for the chair; it is simply a reminder to the speaker that it is time to stop talking and give others the opportunity to speak. If no one shows a desire to speak, it is still beneficial for the group to remain silent for a few moments so that everyone can recover from the concentration given to the previous speaker and think about the direction they wish the discussion to take.

If you are the one who is given a time signal, you have several benefits: You have an opportunity to reassess the direction your lengthy comments were taking and refocus on the group as a whole. If you have become somewhat strident, you can take time to calm down.

Calming the Air

Another hand motion that you can use in face-to-face groups is a calming motion, sometimes using both hands, palm down, moving in a slow, circular motion, as if you were petting a cat. This motion is very helpful for groups that tend to work with a high level of anxiety and stress, or that tend to erupt into unproductive sparking types of discussion. Frequent eruptions with everyone talking at once signals that anxiety and stress are running amok. A group can benefit from recognizing this pattern in their interactions and deliberately choosing to take steps to change what happens.

The calming-the-air motion reminds the group of their commitment to end interactions that feed unproductive anxieties, choosing instead those interactions that help everyone remain focused and calm. When someone calms the air, the group ceases what is happening, takes a deep breath together, and remains still while they gather their thoughts and feelings to address what is going on.

In online groups, a calming signal can be agreed upon by the group. The message can be one or two simple words: "Everyone breathe!" When this message is posted, no further explanation is needed. The group understands that this is a call to remain silent for a few hours, and to resume posts in a spirit of returning to a focus on the group as a whole.

Random Ravings

Sometimes people think of loose ends that were not completely finished during a discussion, or the group leaves a piece of business hanging for lack of clarity on the matter. At some point during a face-to-face gathering, usually toward the end, loose ends tend to become more obvious. It is helpful to set aside a few moments for everyone to reflect on any items that may need to be mentioned briefly before the end of the meeting. This time on the agenda is referred to as "random ravings."[1] Online, you can enter the words "random raving" in the subject line of your message.

While you take notes during the gathering, remember that you can address random ravings later. You can simply circle any note you want to address later and not interrupt the flow of discussion. When the time for random ravings arrives, a quick review of your notes will help you recall these fleeting thoughts. Group members can scan their notes to see if any loose ends might be dangling that now need to be addressed. If a loose end deserves more discussion, the group can agree to place the item on the agenda for the next discussion.

Clusters

Large groups can draw on the processes for Peace and Power, but need to do so using clusters. A large face-to-face gathering can begin with small clusters of participants checking in with one another, followed by each cluster reporting significant information with the large group. For example, if everyone in a cluster is in fine spirits and ready to participate fully in the gathering, then this cluster will simply report this to the group as a whole. If another cluster has a member who is recovering from being sick all week, and who will need to leave early to go to an appointment with the nurse practitioner, this can be shared with the large group. Another cluster might have someone who wants to place a 10-minute presentation on the agenda. Throughout the gathering, the group moves from the whole to clusters and back again.

A large online group can have several clusters, each with their own private e-mail discussion group. Most of their online attention is within the cluster until the structure of the larger group calls for their active participation.

When clusters are used, there is a convener of the whole, and there may also be conveners of the clusters, depending on the needs of the smaller groups. Clusters may need to make a written record of some of their discussions, either to recall the specifics of their work for reporting later to the larger group, or to contribute to a written record of the work of the whole group. When value-based decisions are required, clusters can be a very effective means of making sure that every perspective is considered carefully, with each cluster taking a particular aspect of the decision as a focus for their discussion.

Example 7–1   Online Task Group

A local quilter's club that works to preserve antique quilts and quilting designs, history, and techniques decides that they need to revise their by-laws. Four people volunteer for this task. They set up an online e-mail group so that they can do most of their work from home since they live far apart from one another. The free service for the e-mail group provides them with a Web page where all of their e-mail messages can be archived and where they can upload drafts of the by-laws for everyone to review. They also are able to upload resource material, post links to Web sites that provide important information, and develop a database that could track the progress of each of the tasks they need to accomplish to finish the by-laws revision. They post photographs on their Web page of their quilt projects so that they can become better acquainted with one another and their particular interests.

As they get started with their online discussion of what they need to do and how to go about it, they realize that Annie has not participated in the discussion. Olga calls her on the phone to make sure she is okay and to ask if she is going to be able to continue with the group. Olga finds out that Annie's computer had to go in for repairs, and that she expects to be back online the next day.

Continued

Example 7–1 *continued*

   Once they know Annie is online again, Suzanne summarizes the various suggestions that group members have made
so far and outlines a draft of a plan to revise the by-laws.
Since Olga and Jane have never worked on by-laws before,
Suzanne also provides some online resources to which they
can all refer as guides for how to go about this task. Each person in the group agrees to take on a specific responsibility,
and they all agree on dates to report back to the group what
they have accomplished.

   From time to time, someone posts a question or a request
for assistance online, and the others respond if they are able to
answer the question or give assistance. Their work goes along
smoothly until Jane is hospitalized unexpectedly. Annie, who
lives nearby, visits Jane in the hospital and conveys to the
group that she is going to be okay, but probably will not be
able to work on the project. Since they are almost done with
the revision, they easily adjust the remaining work to be done
and complete everything in the time they had promised.

To Deepen Your Appreciation of the Ideas in This Chapter . . .

   Think about a recent group discussion in which you participated. Did everyone in the group have a chance to speak?
   Did everyone in the group pay attention to what the speaker
   was saying? If so, does this happen because of a rule or
   strong leader who makes sure that discussions go this way?
   Does this happen because everyone in the group is committed to and values having every voice heard? If your group
   discussion does not provide a chance for everyone to speak,
   and if people do not pay attention to one another or talk over
   one another, what do you think would be needed for the
   group to change?

   Try the process of circling in a small, informal group. This
   might be a few members of your family, or friends gathered
   for a meal. Share with the group what you understand about
   circling and why you think it could be useful. Identify with
   the group something that everyone would like to hear everyone talk about—something in which everyone is interested
   and something that does not bring up negative or tense feel-

ings in the group. Be sure that everyone understands that each person is to speak, and that while one person is speaking everyone else is to listen without interruption. If you think it would be helpful, suggest that people make brief notes each time they are tempted to interrupt. Clarify that there will be no open discussion until every person has spoken. Each person can speak until they are done, but remind people to be aware of the time needed for everyone else to speak. Later, reflect on this experience, identify what you liked about the experience and things that you might change. Consider how you might use this process in other situations.

☙ Find an opportunity where you can observe a discussion between two or more people. Notice how often people are interrupted when they are speaking. What happens when someone is interrupted? Does everyone interrupt the others, or do one or two people more often interrupt? How do you feel about what you observe?

☙ Continue your Peace and Power reflections for this chapter. Review your reflections from earlier chapters. What questions or issues are persisting for you as you go through each chapter? Highlight these issues and consider why these are particularly important for you.

Note

1. Anne Montes of Buffalo, New York, suggested the idea of random ravings, and it instantly became a regular part of our gatherings. This is a wonderful example of how the possibilities for Peace and Power processes grow and expand.

CHAPTER 8

VALUE-BASED DECISION-BUILDING

Peace and Power value-based decision-building:

- assures the best decisions that are possible at the time the decisions are made.
- includes flexible options to address different kinds of decisions.
- opens doors to using disagreements to build understanding.
- reduces misunderstandings concerning what the decision means for individuals and for the group.
- nurtures collective memory of the group's values and the path taken to put these values into action.
- brings together different perspectives on a situation, rather than polarizing points of view in opposition to one another.
- nurtures understanding, insight, and wisdom for everyone who participates.

These seemingly idealistic features of group interactions in the processes of forming decisions are possible because of the focus on the quality of the process, as well as the quality of the decisions themselves. As you might expect, groups that utilize Peace and Power decision-building reach decisions in ways that are very different from the practices of traditional hierarchical groups. Some of the practices used in traditional decision-making can be used, but these are used mindfully, based on the nature of the questions the group is asking and the values that members bring to the forefront in forming a decision.

Value-based decision-building uses a comprehensive approach to addressing an issue that combines individual preferences (as in voting), hearing all points of view (as in consensus), and brainstorming all possibilities (as in creative problem solving). In addition, value-based decision-building incorporates processes of values clarification, conflict mediation, critical thinking, and problem solving.

Value-based decision-building within a diverse group is possible because it is formed in the context of the group's purpose, and is built consciously to be consistent with the group's principles of solidarity. At the same time, decision-building processes contribute to clarifying and revising the purpose of the group and the principles of solidarity.

Value-based decisions are stronger, more valuable, and more lasting than those achieved by a majority, where (sometimes large and important) minority preferences are not taken into account. A value-based group decision is also stronger than any decision made is by an individual, no matter how well-informed that individual is. When everyone has participated in building a decision, all individuals can act in concert with that decision because they understand how and why the decision was reached.

Voting, which uses and reinforces a divisive power-over dynamic within groups, is not used in value-based decision-building as a way of making a decision. Instead, the group values and carefully considers all opinions, even if only one person brings a particular opinion to the group. As each perspective is considered, it is integrated as an explicit part of the decision, or as a factor that informs the direction the group takes. The group may often want or need to know how many of its members hold a particular perspective, and so the group may take a straw vote. However, this is for information only, and typically is not the only factor taken into account in building a decision.

Consensus decision-making is quite like value-based decision-building; in fact, previous editions of this book focused on consensus. However, common understandings of consensus do not consciously ground a decision in the values of the group, which is a key element of the kind of decision-building that is central to Peace and Power processes. Consensus, therefore, is defined as any approach to decision-making that focuses on taking into account all perspectives, and finding a perspective that integrates as many of these perspectives as possible. The pitfall of consensus is that the group can flounder without a clear understanding of which direction to take among many choices. A value-based decision-building approach shapes the direction and purpose around which the decision is built.

Value-based decision-building is not to be confused with compromise. Compromise requires that each person give something up in accepting a decision. Compromise decision-making is often called consensus decision-making simply because the group is not voting, but instead trying to agree. True consensus decision-making does incorporate the process of exploring fully all options and finding the best option for the group, whereas compromise decision-making involves finding that upon which all individuals can agree. In seeking simply to achieve agreement, the group relies on individuals making concessions that result in a bottom line on which everyone can agree—often a weak and unsatisfactory outcome for the group. In contrast, value-based decision-building embraces differences of individual perspectives while building solidarity around the group's purposes.

Value-based decision-building starts with the benefits the group envisions, so that it is a process that focuses on what each person and the group as a whole gain by the nature of the decision they reach. The group carefully considers individual's wishes, preferences, or desires, and integrates these in light of the group's shared purposes. Each individual shifts attention to that which the group as a whole sincerely values as a community. If an individual concedes a personal preference, it is done as an affirmative step to collectively support the group's shared purpose and vision.

Value-based decision-building is not totalitarian group-think. What protects against this is the commitment to hear and value all points of view, and to refrain from bringing closure until all possibilities have been addressed fully. The group's principles of solidarity provide the common focus for examining diverse views, but are a guide, not dogma. A new viewpoint on an issue can challenge the group to re-examine their principles of solidarity, resulting in healthy growth and change.

A common concern when you first consider value-based decision-building is that the process will be time consuming and inefficient. It does take more time to reach a decision using value-based decision-building. However, groups that shift to this approach almost never have to retrace their decision, nor do they have to spend time making sure that everyone is on the same page. It is not possible to determine the time and effort saved when everyone understands the decision and fully supports the decision, but to take shortcuts in building a decision is a sure setup for wasted time and frustration later. The overall benefits of cohesiveness, acting in accord together rather than at cross purposes, and mutual understanding more than compensate for the time invested in reaching a decision in this manner.

How the Process Works

The process of value-based decision-building is deliberate and thoughtful. It is a process very well-suited to online interactions, ideally as a complement to face-to-face discussions. Having the ability to take some of your discussion online gives a permanent record of your deliberations for future reference, keeps everyone informed of facts and resources that the group used in reaching a decision, and reinforces the value of each person taking time to consider the perspectives of everyone in the group.

Value-based decision-building includes the following processes that typically unfold in the following sequence, but that also can be used in fluid and circular patterns.

- Pose the central question or questions toward which the decision is oriented. For example, "Should we look for another location for our Center?" "What kind of programs should we offer in the coming year?" "Where should we meet?" While this seems to be a simple step, it is often overlooked, and groups set about trying to make decisions with many different perspectives concerning what the decision really is about.
- Explore which of your principles of solidarity are central to this question. If a group has a principle of solidarity that sets forth a commitment to work within a specific budget, and not to place strain on that budget, then when they approach the issue of finding a new location, their process of decision-building needs to be guided by this principle. Or, the group may come to realize that they need to stretch the limits of what might be possible beyond the constraints of the budget as they now see it in order to achieve certain goals that they also value highly. If your group has not yet formed principles of solidarity, take time to identify together the values that you all agree are the most important in guiding this decision.
- Describe the benefits that the group envisions for any decision that arises from this process. These benefits reflect underlying values that the group uses as yardsticks against which to measure the soundness of various options. These benefits need to be consistent with the group's central principles of solidarity, but they are more situation-specific to the decision at hand. For example, a group that is contemplating a new location might identify the following benefits of any new location: it must be accessible to people who are underserved; it must remain

within their budget; and it must provide the kind of space that is required to implement a new program that the group wishes to begin.

- Brainstorm as many different perspectives on the question as possible. At this point, be clear that every possibility is open for discussion. No decision is contemplated or implied in this process. Remain open to all possibilities, even if they seem ludicrous at the time.

- Use whatever means are indicated to gather the information needed to inform the decision. Obtain factual data, consult others in the community, or bring in guests to provide specialized information. Find out what has happened to other groups in similar circumstances. If at any time the group wants to know how many prefer one option over others, pause to take a straw vote that gives everyone information about where people stand on the issue at this point in time. Votes are not taken to decide an issue, but rather to inform the deliberation. After the group votes, take the time to have people speak to why they favor one option over others.

- As you reach a point where you have considered many possibilities and you have before you all the information you can gather, begin to weigh the most viable options seriously against the benefits you set forth early in the process. Narrow the possibilities to those options that are most congruent with these benefits.

- If none of the options seems fully adequate, and the decision is one that cannot be set aside, then shift to consider how the group can move forward. Discuss the feasibility of moving forward with the option that seems the best at this time. Discuss as well what needs are not met if you take this direction, and how the group can make provisions to address these needs in the future.

The most difficult challenge in value-based decision-building is determining in advance the benefits the group seeks in making a decision. However, once the group settles upon this common ground, reaching a sound decision becomes a relatively smooth process. The group can see directions that clearly will lead to a good and sound decision that takes into account—but is not dominated by—individual preferences.

Table 8–1 illustrates the links between the question that gives a focus to a decision and the benefits that might be envisioned and the key processes that the group uses in building a decision.

TABLE 8–1   Questions, Benefits, and Key Decision-Building Processes

Question	What Benefits Do We Seek?	Key Decision-Building Processes
Where should we meet next year? (Options are scattered around the continental United States and Canada)	The majority of our members need to be present.	Honor the preference of the majority, making sure that a significant number of those will, in fact, be able to attend.
	Members who have particular knowledge and skill in the area of political processes need to be present, along with as many others as possible.	Consider the preference of the majority in light of the preferences of those members with the needed knowledge and skills.
	Location needs to provide low cost for members, child care, accessibility, etc. In order to make the meeting accessible to many who would not otherwise be able to attend.	Gather information about key sites that are possible and use this information to inform the decision. Make sure that the provisions are sufficient to assure participation from those who might not otherwise be able to attend.
	All of the above are equally important benefits.	Review all of the information required for each benefit and use this to guide making the best decision possible.

Example 8–1   Location

Consider the dilemma of a group that is considering a new location because the lease on their current space is not being renewed. They do not have the option to stay where they are. They have agreed that any new location must be accessible to people who are underserved; it must remain within their budget; and it must provide the kind of space that is required to implement a new program that the group wishes to begin.

There is one location that would be accessible and that provides adequate space, but the cost is greater than their budget. Five of the twenty members of the group favor this

Question	What Benefits Do We Seek?	Key Decision-Building Processes
What should be included on the program for next year's International Women's Day celebration?	We must work within our budget.	Gather information regarding costs of possible program features, and decide based on what can fit within the budget.
	It is important to present a diverse program, and then raise the money to do it.	Bring together all ideas for the program and select a profile that represents the greatest diversity. Determine what is required for funding, and set this as the goal for fund-raising.
	We need to reach women in the community who are alienated and underrecognized.	Bring together voices of women you seek to reach and plan the program based on what they convey is important to them.
	We need to reach underrecognized women, but must also work within our budget.	Decide based on what women convey is important to them, and together review how these features can be addressed within the budget you have.

space and wish to move forward and find a way to make up the difference in the cost. The other option is a space that is within the budget and accessible, but that does not provide the needed space. Fifteen of the members favor this space.

As the group continues to discuss their options, everyone agrees that not to move forward with the new program would be shortsighted, particularly since within 18 months the new program will bring in new income. They turn their attention to figuring out how they might address the budget issue, and two of those who initially "voted" against this option find a grant that can cover the deficit until the new program begins to bring in new income. They apply for the grant, it is awarded, and the group contracts for the larger space.

Calling for Closure

When the group has considered all points of view about an issue, the convener or another member of the group summarizes what may be the predominant sense of the group and asks if this summary is satisfactory to all who are present. At this point, any alternate viewpoint is expressed and the discussion continues with a focus on reaching a conclusion that takes into account all viewpoints. When there are no new possibilities, the group has built a decision.

Although the process at times seems unending by encouraging full discussion of controversy and differences, the satisfaction that comes from being clear about the values and benefits the group seeks, and from hearing each individual's thoughts and ideas, far outweighs any frustrations. Although the process seems tedious, value-based decision-building is often more efficient than other forms of decision-making. This is true because there is rarely misunderstanding about what the group has decided, and people can invest fully in acting on the decision.

If discussion of an issue does not flow easily to build a decision, the group can decide not to decide and leave the issue open for later discussion. Actually, there are few decisions that are truly urgent. Having to decide not to decide carries its own message: More thought and planning needs to go into the matter to form a sound decision.

If a decision seems urgent and the group is unable to reach closure, someone needs to call for the group to reflect on how urgent the decision really is. If it is truly not urgent, or if they can make an interim decision, the group leaves the matter open and places it on the agenda for the next gathering. If the decision is urgent, then the group must focus on the necessity of reaching a decision that everyone can live with for now, and plan for more discussion of the issues involved. Even in this circumstance, the more that the group is able to identify the values upon which the decision is built, the more satisfactory the decision will be in the long run.

Every member does not need to be present in a face-to-face group whenever the group makes a decision. In online-only groups, it is seldom that someone has to be absent from the decision-building process. If your group combines online interaction with face-to-face discussion, you can ensure that everyone in the group is likely to be equally informed and capable of contributing to the decision. If you are not able to have everyone involved in reaching a decision, those who are present can reach closure because the group's principles of solidarity guide the process. However, if the decision being considered is one that directly affects the work of members of the group who are not present, consider the decision as tentative until all individuals who are affected can be part of the discussion. If those who are not present bring new viewpoints to the matter, then the group continues the discussion over several gatherings to assure that everyone has the opportunity to participate as much as possible in the discussion and in the decision-building process.

Positive Dissent

Dissent occurs when the group is close to reaching closure in the decision-building process, and one or more people indicate that they still have serious concerns and are not ready to reach closure. The right of an individual or small minority to dissent is a strength that guards against the dangers of totalitarian group think. In order to assure that dissent proceeds as a positive strength in the decision-building process, consider the following specific questions when you face dissent in building a value-based decision.[1]

- Have those who are dissenting fully disclosed their objections, and the underlying concerns, values, and reasons for their objections? Everyone may need to help in placing words around an individual's concerns. Sometimes getting clear about exactly what is motivating dissent is not an easy thing to do, especially when you are in the difficult situation of being alone in your opinion. If you are in the majority, you may not agree with those who are dissenting. Take care not to assume that the dissenters have fully disclosed their concerns. Turn your attention to helping to find a way to express and understand their underlying concerns.

- Have all members of the group fully heard, and do we all appreciate the concerns of those dissenting? One way to affirm the group's solidarity in appreciation of the minority view is to ask each person to state the dissent in her or his own way, and reflect to the group what she or he might do if this were her or his own perspective. In other words, have everyone place themselves in the shoes of those who hold the dissenting view. When you strongly disagree with the dissenting point of view, remember that in expressing something you disagree with you are seeking to understand it, not necessarily to agree with it. By remaining sincerely committed to understanding another point of view, you contribute to building a decision that brings people together, rather than puts them at odds with one another.

- What underlying principle of solidarity or value does this situation bring to light? The value or principle may not be one that the group has addressed before, and getting clear about a new underlying value can have a major influence on what next step the group takes. If you identify an underlying value that is already part of your group's principles, and this situation is challenging that value, this is a signal that the group may be at a turning point in its growth.

- What are all the possible decisions that we could make on this issue, taking into account this dissenting perspective? Which of these possible decisions could best reflect our group's purpose and our principles of solidarity? Once you have all the alternatives clearly identified and once you explicitly match the alternatives with what your group is really all about, you may be able to reach closure.

If your group considers these questions and they lead to productive discussion, you are experiencing positive and growth-encouraging dissent. If instead you become more confused and alienated from one another, then you are likely to be embroiled in a divisive power struggle. Despite the positive potential of dissent, dissenting individuals hold enormous potential to act in a divisive power-over manner. If you find yourself in a situation that cannot be resolved, you and the group have special responsibilities to carefully consider exactly what is happening.

Reaching a point in the decision-building process where positions are polarized is a signal that the group as a whole needs to step away from the "what" of the discussion and examine underlying values and commitments. To do this, move to processes for conflict transformation (Chapter 10). When most people in the group want to settle the matter and get on with things, it can feel very tedious to shift into a process of conflict transformation. However, when you consider the typical alternatives—hurt feelings, misunderstandings beyond repair, broken relationships, the resentment and anger that grow from unresolved disagreement—taking the time to attend to what is happening in the group is an attractive alternative indeed!

Example 8–2   Deciding When to Meet

The following example illustrates the differences between compromise decision-making (where the focus is on what individuals have to concede) and value-based decision-building (where the focus is on what everyone and the group gains). The decision—when to meet—seems on the surface like a relatively easy and somewhat inconsequential decision. However, this decision, like any other, calls on and reveals the values and strengths of the group in building community. It also illustrates how a relatively simple matter can be used as an occasion for the group to practice decision-building skills, so that as more weighty decisions come before the group, everyone has experienced the processes and understands what is happening.

In this example, a group of students in a very intensive program have formed a support group to study together and to practice the skills they are learning in a safe and supportive context. The demands of their class schedules and personal lives make it very difficult to find a mutually convenient time to meet, but all members of the group remain adamant that they want to meet weekly. They all agree that the purpose of meeting weekly is to assist one another in learning new skills, and that the benefits of meeting as a group are essential to their individual well-being and success in the program. They agree that they are "all in this together," and want to make the commitment to contribute to one another's success in the program by getting together weekly to practice.

After some discussion, the group decides to circle to be clear about everyone's preference. Several prefer Wednesday mid-day during a 90-minute break between classes. Several others prefer Friday afternoon after class. Those who object to Wednesday believe that cramming a group meeting between two long classes makes the day too long and intense. Those who object to Friday believe that they are too burned out at the end of classes on Friday to be able to participate in the group, and several have family or job responsibilities at this time.

Sue: How about if we rotate days? Then people could participate on the days they prefer.

Sally: Then we would really be breaking into two separate groups. I would rather not do that.

Continued

Example 8–2 *continued*

> *Randy:* Wait a minute. I suggested a possibility—to meet before class on Wednesdays, when we are all fresh and not tired. Nobody has paid any attention to what I suggested.

The group decides to circle again to make sure that everyone has considered Randy's suggestion, and to see if people have any other new ideas. People comment on the possible benefits of meeting before class on Wednesday, but just about everyone objects to starting the day very early in the morning (7:00 a.m.) and then being in class until 4:30 in the afternoon.

> *Amanda:* Well, it seems to me that most people have spoken in favor of Friday. After all, we will never find a time that suits everyone. Can we just agree to meet Friday for at least six weeks, and then change to another time if people want to do that?

Resigned, everyone agrees. In this scenario, the group has actually voted based on the majority favoring Friday as the meeting time. In reality, most of the people who expressed support for Friday also have reservations about the meeting time, and share the concerns of many who favored Wednesday. Those who favored Wednesday will, of necessity, be left out of participating on Friday because of their other commitments on Friday. Nobody leaves feeling particularly good. What is missing at this point is a real focus on the purpose and benefits that they agreed upon early in their discussion of a meeting time. The group did not integrate this as a key element in the decision-building process. They are caught in a conflict of wills, where individual preference is the only factor that was taken into consideration.

On the next Friday, the group meets and everyone is present, with many making personal sacrifices to be there. During check-in, several people make clear to the group how tired they are and how much they wish they could find another time to meet. The agenda was supposed to focus on planning several practice sessions before the mid-term exams. Amanda tells the group she has thought about the time-to-meet issue, and wants to at least share some of her thoughts before they start the agenda.

> *Amanda:* Look, I don't necessarily want to open this thing up again, so if people don't want to discuss this after I

tell you my thoughts I will be okay with that. But I was thinking that we need to shift our focus to why we want to do this in the first place—which is to be a support group for one another. We clearly can't all always be here for lots of different reasons, even when we want to be. We just don't want to meet at a time that blocks someone from being able to be here (like when they have to be at work). So what I am wondering is, how can we be a support group for one another but not depend exclusively on when we meet? For example, we have a phone tree. We could use that to pass along words of encouragement and funny jokes—not just announcements about snow days! We could also look at the time we meet in light of when during the week we are feeling the most vulnerable and in need of support. I think it would be very supportive if we know when the group meets and where, and what is going to be happening, so if I want to consider not being there I know what I am missing, and I can always connect with folks who can be there.

Jo: What you are saying makes so much sense, Amanda, and it does fit with something I thought about after our last discussion. I was so turned off by that whole thing that I really began to wonder what kind of support we could be for one another if we can't even decide about when to meet and feel good about what we decided. I was just totally wiped out after that meeting, and all I could think about was what on earth went wrong.

Sue: I agree. After our last discussion, I realized that I really don't like the idea of rotating the days like I had suggested. Sally was right in pointing out that then we would break into two groups. I think that having a regular day and time is important because this leaves no question about how to find one another and where, when we really do need to connect.

Sally: Another thing I think is important is what Amanda said: We all need to know what is going to happen from week to week so we can decide if it is worth being there. I want this group to be meaningful and important—not just a feel-good party time,

Continued

Example 8–2   *continued*

>   although I hope we party some! But if I am really
>   tired or stressed out, I need to know what the group
>   is planning to do to make a good decision about
>   whether to make the effort to be there.
> *Randy:*   What if only one or two people show up and they
>   really need other people there to help with their
>   practice, but the rest of us have decided that it is
>   not worth our effort to be there?

Everyone pauses while people think about this possibility.

> *Stephanie:*   We could agree that if anyone is going to the meet-
>   ing knowing they need to practice, and they need
>   others there to give feedback, then let all of us
>   know in class so that the rest of us can realize how
>   important this is to someone, and plan to go to help
>   one another if we can possibly do it. After all, to
>   me that is what support means: helping one another
>   and not just getting help for myself. But it would
>   also help me if I know what my friends need.
> *Melanie:*   And I do want our time to be productive and worth-
>   while. I will be very motivated to be there even at a
>   time that is inconvenient for me if I am sure we are
>   all committed to making it worthwhile.

Everyone pauses again. This time the pause suggests that
they have no additional viewpoints to share.

> *Amanda:*   I've been taking some notes. Here's what I have so
>   far. We need a stable time and place for the group
>   to meet so we can plan ahead. Everyone needs to
>   know in advance what the topic or activity is going
>   to be. We want to know any individual needs
>   before the group meets, when this is possible. We
>   want to make it productive and worthwhile time in
>   terms of supporting one another. Anything else
>   so far?

The group affirms Amanda's summary and makes a few
suggestions to refine it. They then decide that they will stay with
the Friday time. After all, they were all able to shift their other
responsibilities to be here today (even though this will not
always be possible). They decide to reassess the time of their

meetings at the end of the term, and more importantly, to reflect on how they are feeling about their ability to support one another. They agree that everyone needs to be present for that discussion, and everyone indicates a willingness to make that commitment. Stephanie agrees to convene the next meeting and to circulate an initial draft of a plan for practicing so that they can discuss the plan quickly next Friday, and begin practicing their skills to make good use of their time together.

Example 8-3   Online Value-Based Decision-Building

A group of lesbian nurses has been organized for several years and only meets online; they are scattered in several countries, and their primary focus is to provide support and resources for one another as they deal with the challenges of being lesbian. Tracy in Canada sends a message to the group that she is exploring the idea of a project to interview lesbian nurses and compile their stories into a publication of some sort. She asks if the group would be interested in taking this on as a group project, or if people think she should do this on her own. Everyone who responds is delighted with the idea, and they encourage her to share more details about what she envisions this project to be. No one volunteers to help take on the task, but there is a general sense that the group would like for this to be a group effort.

Tracy posts a more detailed proposal, and a few people send messages saying it looks great, or giving some minor suggestions for editing. Jo notices that the group has not really responded to Tracy's question about the group taking this on as a group task. So Jo posts a message that puts the question to the group: "Should we as a group take on the project that Tracy has described?" She asks the group to post messages that give their sense of how well this project would address their purposes of providing support and resources for lesbian nurses, and how well this project would benefit the group. She also asks everyone to post something within the next two weeks if possible. Jo also asks for someone in the group to volunteer to summarize the discussion at the end of the two weeks. Brandy and Janet both volunteer to do this.

Continued

Example 8–3   *continued*

At the end of the two weeks, Brandy and Janet both post their summaries of the discussion. Their summaries turn out to be very interesting; they are both enthusiastic about and supportive of the project, but Brandy's summary tended to focus on the group's purposes, and Janet's focused on how the project could benefit the group. It seemed clear that everyone felt the project is badly needed as a resource, as well as for supportive affirmation of lesbian existence in nursing, benefiting not only members of the group but all lesbian nurses now and in the future. Several people in the group noted how important the project would be for nurses who are not lesbians, as a way to bring about a better understanding between those who are and those who are not lesbians.

Brandy's summary brought out a minority point of view in the discussion—that to take on such a project would detract the group from the more personal, day-to-day and spontaneous support that the online group provided. She noted that several people felt that if the e-mail messages started focusing on getting a job done, they would become turned off and could easily tune out what was going on. They feared they would lose the sense of turning to the e-mail group to learn about day-to-day challenges that lesbian nurses face, and being able to reach out on a more personal level of communication to provide encouragement, support and assistance.

What followed were several days of discussion, with many saying that they had not considered the effect this project would have on the group, and feeling quite strongly that they did not want the nature of the group to shift in this way. By the end of the fifth day, Jo sent a message summarizing what she sensed was the general conclusion of the group, that the group supported Tracy's idea and wanted it to go forward, but that it should not be a task for the e-mail group to take on. She called for the group to "e-circle" to determine how much consensus they really had. Everyone posted a brief message summarizing her own opinion, with all agreeing that the project should go forward but not as a group project. Several individuals volunteered then to work with Tracy, and they formed another online group to proceed with the project.

To Deepen Your Appreciation of the Ideas in This Chapter . . .

> Recall a decision that your group made recently. Was this decision consistent with the values of the group? How was the decision made? Was everyone satisfied with the decision? If some people were not satisfied and others were, can you fully express each point of view involved?

> Consider a time when you have disagreed with the majority of others in your group about a decision the group was making. What happened when you expressed your point of view? Did the group take your opinion into account? What did the group do, or what could they have done to fully appreciate your point of view?

> Find an opportunity to observe a group making a decision using typical voting and Robert's Rules of Order. Do you see ways in which the group is already using one or more of the processes used in value-based decision-building? For example, does the group brainstorm different possibilities, or do they identify the benefits they envision for this decision? What would be required for this group to fully shift to value-based decision building, and how would the group benefit by doing so?

> Continue your Peace and Power reflections for this chapter. Review your reflections from earlier chapters. Did you have earlier questions that are becoming clearer as you reflect on this chapter?

Note

1. The Center for Conflict Resolution book entitled *Building United Judgment: A Handbook for Consensus Decision Making* (1981) provides an excellent in-depth discussion of the processes, possibilities, and challenges of consensus decision-making. These questions are informed by many of their suggestions and insights.

CHAPTER 9

CLOSING

Closing is:

- reflecting on the group's effectiveness.
- gaining self-knowledge and knowledge of the group.
- strengthening communication within the group.
- focusing on how you have interacted rather than what you have done.
- expressing love and respect for individuals and the group.

Closing is a time when all members share thoughts and feelings about what has happened, and about what they would like to happen next. Each individual's closing is a three-part statement that includes the following:

- appreciation for someone or something that has happened during the process of your time together,
- critical reflection that brings to the group constructive insights about the processes of the group, *and*
- affirmation that expresses commitment to moving forward with the group's work and individual growth.

Closing a gathering or an online discussion using this process *ensures* that the group remains open to envisioning and exploring alternatives and uses the experiences of the group to form the future. Closing is a process that brings each individual's intent and commitment together with the group's principles of solidarity. The overall purpose of closing is to strengthen the group and each individual.

Although closing is one of the most important, rewarding, and beneficial of the Peace and Power processes, it is hard to take the time and energy needed to do it. Often groups get caught up in what they are doing and forget to set aside the brief time needed at the end to reflect on how they have interacted together. Closing is not always easy to do and initially can feel risky. During closing, feelings that were simply undercurrents during discussion may be expressed openly, something that is not customary in typical groups. Ironically, feelings of caring and appreciation are also usually not expressed openly in groups. Angry or hurt feelings are especially avoided because they are simply not supposed to be acknowledged openly. During closing, group members acknowledge their feelings in constructive ways so that everyone in the group can develop a fuller understanding of one another and of the group. When this happens, everyone has the benefit of knowing what is really going on, internally for individuals and within the group. Every time your group practices the skills involved in closing, you are building an important foundation for the skills of conflict transformation (Chapter 10).

Closing Processes

Use closing to end gatherings, to end a lengthy or intense discussion on a single topic, or to signal a transition in an online discussion from one time frame to another. When the time to close arrives, set discussion aside and shift focus to reflection on the group's process. To have the benefit of closing, everyone who has participated in the gathering or the online discussion needs to be fully present for closing.

Sometimes you may be tempted to skip closing, especially in the early stages of getting established, or when decision-building has consumed your time. This is unwise, because closing is a process that ensures that you and the group maintain the habits and practices that make Peace and Power values real. Once you begin to experience the benefits of closing, your group will become very dedicated to setting aside the time you need for closing.

One way to estimate the time you need in a face-to-face group is to plan for each person to have a few seconds to speak during closing. Or, for a 1-hour meeting, plan about 10 minutes for closing. For a gathering of a day or longer, set aside a half hour or so for closing. At the agreed-upon time, the group takes a few minutes for each person to silently reflect on what has happened during the discussion and to review notes about the gathering. People then share their appreciation, critical reflection, and affirmation.

Closing is as important and as effective in online groups as it is in face-to-face groups. The main difference is that any component of closing can be communicated at any time by any participant, without interrupting the flow of a discussion. If the online group has a structure for their interactions based on periods of time, they may agree to post their complete closing messages at a particular time. For example, if the group's discussion focuses on a topic a week, the group might ask everyone to post their check-in on Monday, and their closing message on Friday.

Appreciation

Appreciation acknowledges something that someone did or said, or a positive group interaction. It is a brief but meaningful statement. This is a time to nurture one another actively by sharing your ideas about specific ways in which you and the group benefited from something that happened. For example, if someone's comment in the discussion was a turning point to help clarify an issue for you, or moved the group discussion to a different level, you might state your appreciation for the comment, and share with the group how or why this comment was so important to you and the group.

Appreciation includes the following elements:

- the names of individuals who are responsible for what it is you appreciate
- a brief description of their specific acts or behavior
- sharing what this means to you as an individual within the group
- your ideas about what this means in terms of the group's purposes or principles of solidarity

Appreciation might be stated in this way: "I appreciate your leadership, Amanda, in shifting our focus from our individual wants and needs to our collective purpose. I learned so much by what you did and how that turned our discussion into working so well together."

Critical Reflection

Critical reflection is careful, precise, thoughtful insight directed toward transformation. It is a tool for becoming aware of actions and behaviors that maintain an unjust society. It flourishes as a positive group process when everyone understands that your collective intention is to support one another in a constructive way, and when you consistently treat one another respectfully. When you use critical reflection with commitment to Peace and Power values, you practice a powerful skill to move toward agreement on what will be done and why. By working through disagreements and doubts, a group is better able to remain cohesive and can continue to work together when the going gets tough.

Critical reflection is like criticism in the arts, where developing your art to its finest level depends upon your own and others' constructive criticism. The practice of Peace and Power is an art form that you create and refine each time you engage with your group. Critical reflection deepens your appreciation of the group and your work and reveals what creative possibilities can develop further.

An art critic brings to the art insights and interpretations that help others to appreciate more fully what the artist has done and what the art means for the culture as a whole. The critic does not proclaim the "correct" view of the art, but does provide a well-informed, knowledgeable interpretation of the art that helps others understand the art better, even if they do not agree with the views of the critic.

In Peace and Power processes, your critical reflection brings to the group the best that you have to offer with the intent of helping everyone in the group better understand what the group is all about. Frame your critical reflection so that you claim ownership of your concerns, provide specific and clear content, and do so in a way that is likely to be heard and received by others in the group.[1]

A constructive critical reflection that encourages and supports growth includes these components.

- "I feel . . ." (your own feeling about what has happened)
- "When (or about) . . . " (a specific action, behavior, or circumstance that is the focus of your thinking)
- "I want . . ." (specific changes you want to happen)
- "Because . . ." (how your concern connects with the group's principles of solidarity)

A closing critical reflection typically calls for a response from others at a later time. Your concern might be addressed apart from the group's gatherings or placed on a future agenda for discussion. Here are two examples:

- "I feel anxious about the fact that we skipped our discussion to plan for the new member gathering next week. I would like at least four of us to meet either after this meeting or tomorrow to plan for next week and to connect online to refine our plan. We are committed to modeling competence and confidence in our work together, and this is especially important when we are presenting our group to possible new members. Sue, Jen, and Amanda—would you, or anyone else, be willing to work with me on this?"

- "I sensed the tension when we discussed the purchase of a new computer for the office, but we did not acknowledge this and discuss it. We have a commitment to explore issues like this fully and openly, and so I would like to place this on next week's agenda for discussion."

Affirmation

The conclusion of the three-step process of closing is a statement of affirmation that gives the group a sense of the ways in which you are working to grow as an individual and as a member of the group. Affirmations are simple statements that speak to your deeper self. They concentrate your energy on the healing, growth-supporting aspects of your work with the group. They are powerful tools for creating change and growth in a direction that you desire.[2]

An affirmation reflects something that is not yet fully a part of your life, but you state it as if it has already happened. For example, at a time when you feel uncertain about a decision, your affirmation might be: "I trust my own inner sense and the wisdom of our group." When a conflict has disturbed you, an affirmation to help transform the conflict might be: "I reside in the care that we have for each other."[3]

Affirmations offered during closing grow out of your experiences in the group, and often relate to your specific appreciations and critical reflections. Affirmations can also grow out of internal work that you do apart from the group and your experiences in the group. This work involves shifting your attention away from frustrations and problems to possibilities for growth and change. As you reflect on these possibilities, you will begin to form affirmations that provide a message to your inner consciousness that you are receptive to the energy of change moving in a creative, healing direction.

Because your inner consciousness is responsive to repetition, repeat affirmations to yourself, using the same wording again and again, with shifts in the wording as you find what is most comfortable for you. Repeat the affirmations while you are doing rhythmic activities, such as exercising, cleaning, or walking. When you reenter the group, you will bring with you the deep inner resources that you have developed within yourself to participate more effectively in the group.

Initially you may find it difficult to affirm yourself. Until you are comfortable creating your own, use an affirmation that someone else suggests. (See the suggestions below.) As your sense of self-affirmation grows, you will create your own. As you become accustomed to using affirmations as a source of directing your energy to create change, you will become skilled at expressing an affirmation during closing that moves you and the group from the circumstances of the present into a future you choose and create.

The following characterize an affirmation:

- It is a positive, simple, "I" statement.
- It is stated in the present tense.
- It is grounded in your present reality, but also provides a bridge to the future you seek.

Here are some examples:

- I value the light and clarity that I bring to situations.[4]
- All that I know is available to me when I need it.
- I believe in myself and our group.
- I care for my Self.
- I am at peace with those I love.
- I am in tune with my intuition.
- I believe in the power of our group.
- I act with confidence in my ability.
- The love we share for each other nourishes me.
- I willingly release the old and welcome the new in my life.
- I choose wisely because I listen to my inner voice.
- I gladly accept the support of those with whom I work.
- My love for myself brings love and support to all my relationships.

Getting Your Head and Heart Together

Getting ready to participate in closing requires thoughtful reflection so that you are clear about the content of what you want to say before you speak. Once you are clear about the content of your three-part closing statement, you can state it briefly and simply.

You have probably not learned to share your own responses to situations while you are in the situation. If this is the case, do not worry—you are not alone. Doing so does not come easily or naturally. Practice is important. Even more important is a supportive, aware group that is fully committed to each member's growth.

Personal notes that you have taken throughout a discussion are very important at the time of closing. Productive gatherings are rarely uneventful, and in the intensity of the discussion you are likely to have thoughts and feelings about what happened and how it happened. Perhaps your perspective has shifted now that the discussion has ended. You may have become aware of an insight and are reaching a new understanding as the discussion comes to a close. Your notes provide words and ideas that you write as these things happen so that you will not forget, and you can review your inner process when it is time to close. To help clarify or refine your thoughts, ask yourself:

- Did I do what I know? Were my behaviors consistent with my values and with our principles of solidarity?
- Were my actions honestly motivated by love and respect for myself, others, and the group?
- Did I remain alert and aware during discussion, or did I check out mentally at some point?
- Am I aware of conflicts or differences that we still need to address?
- What occurred that promoted my own individual growth and the growth of the group?
- What changes in myself would I like to make?[5]

Responding to Closing

Often what people share during closing requires no immediate response. If something very emotional or heavy comes up during closing, the most important response from the group is to acknowledge what has been shared, clarify to make sure everyone understands the message, and assure that the concerns will be addressed in time.

In face-to-face interactions, you often sense right away if something you say or do during closing creates a confusion or misunderstanding. But online, your closing message can be misunderstood with no easy way to know how the message was received. Peace and Power closing messages call for careful reflection, for mindful attention to what you say, and for full disclosure of your thoughts and feelings. This level of disclosure is not something people are generally accustomed to sharing, but it is essential in written, virtual messages that lack non-verbal clues and direct interaction. In an online group, you have the advantage of taking the time you need to compose your closing carefully, reflect on what you want to say and how you want to say it, and to connect your thoughts and feelings with the group's purposes and principles of solidarity.

Once everyone has completed closing, everyone takes ownership for making any responses open and clear, rather than hidden. The most difficult thing to learn about both appreciation and critical reflection is how to accept them! Hearing statements of appreciation or critical reflection is not easy, especially in front of a group, no matter how skillfully they are delivered.

As you receive the appreciation and critical reflections of others, you have the following responsibilities:

- Remain attentive; listen or read carefully. Do not interrupt or respond impulsively.
- If what you hear is welcome and appreciated, a simple thank-you is sufficient, saving your more enthusiastic response until after the group meeting. Keep the focus on the person who has expressed appreciation and resist any temptation to detract from the growth-encouraging intention of a positive closing.
- If what you receive is difficult to take in, or if you have a different viewpoint to share, let the group know how you feel and be sure the issue is placed on an agenda for a future discussion. Refer to Chapter 10 to ground your thoughts and feelings in the constructive values that the group shares.
- Keep any response to a minimum so that you do not drag out a meeting or online discussion past the time it is supposed to end. Remember that almost everything can wait.

Critical Reflection as Homework

Sometimes you cannot think clearly and speak or write artfully at the time of closing. Often, people can only do so after some time has passed. This gives you the opportunity to do your own internal work at home, especially when it comes to critical reflection. If you sense during a meeting that there is a critical reflection you need to develop on your own, during closing describe the nature of your concern, and ask the group to wait for a fuller discussion later, either during check-in or as an agenda item.

Artful critical reflection arises from your deepest inner awareness, is energized by your emotions, and is finely crafted by your clearest thinking. It is shared with others in a manner and at a time when you can call upon full awareness (including thoughts and feelings) to address the issue.

The homework required to do this includes getting in touch with the full range of feelings that you experience around the issue and thinking about all of the facts and circumstances that are a part of the situation. It requires thinking through similar circumstances that you have experienced to search for a perspective that comes from that broader experience and envisioning future possibilities that might emerge from this experience.

Constructive critical reflection is placed in the context of the purposes of the group. One way to do this is to take time to review the group's principles of solidarity. Think about the present situation in light of each principle and how addressing the issue you are studying can strengthen the group.

Weigh carefully many possibilities. Imagine what might be different in a similar circumstance in the future and possibilities for what might now emerge from the situation as it is. Think about how you and the group might move forward in a direction that you choose carefully rather than a direction that just happens.

As you reflect on the situation, write down ideas and thoughts. You can go over these notes to sort out which of your ideas are beneficial and constructive and rethink ideas that may not be constructive. Once you see your ideas on paper, you can explore different ways of saying things and make sure everything you need to say is there. When you share your ideas with the group, the notes you prepare at home can help you to remain focused and include your full range of feelings and thoughts stated in constructive and beneficial ways.

Example 9-1   Online closing

An online group has decided to start using the process of closing because they realize that there have been too many misunderstandings of one another. It all started when Jeri sent a message to the group saying that she was sick and tired of all the personal stuff that people were sending to the group—it is creating too much e-mail, and she does not want to read all of the details; she is concerned about what is going on with everyone but does not think the group should have detailed personal exchanges on the list. She concluded with saying: "Would people stop doing this so we can get on with things?"

Indeed, there had been a lot of personal messages exchanged in the group. Sandy loved to send jokes to everyone. Kate had found a new recipe to share. Lynne sent pictures

Continued

Example 9–1   *continued*

of her new granddaughter just about every week. Recently, Nora and Jill had both undergone breast biopsies, and when they shared what was happening, everyone responded to let them know they were concerned and would keep them in their thoughts and prayers, offering support and assistance. Kate needed to find a new job and had asked the group for leads. Sally was planning a trip to Guatemala. When Jeri's message came to the group, there were a few hurt feelings, many of them unacknowledged to the group.

Rose, who had sent a number of messages to the group about travel in Guatemala, had recently learned about the Peace and Power process of closing in a class she was taking. She sent a message to the group that drew on what she had learned about closing, and asked the group to consider using this process to avoid having similar misunderstandings in the future. Rose's message stated: "I appreciate everyone in the group participating actively in our discussions, and I appreciate you, Jeri, for bringing up the issue of personal exchanges in our group. I also realize that what you said created some hurt feelings, even though I know you did not intend to be hurtful. And, even though I myself do not share your sense that the personal messages have been too much, I suspect that others do share your feeling about this. I know that we are fully committed to staying focused on what we are doing together, but that we also agree that we want to know one another on a personal level. I would like for everyone in the group to send us a message with ideas as to how we can balance our work and our personal interactions so that we can come up with some guidelines for how to do this. And, I would like us to consider using closing messages regularly so that we address this kind of issue constructively in the future."

It turned out that most of the people in the group did not agree with Jeri that the personal exchanges had been too much, and many appreciated knowing what was going on with everyone else. But they also agreed that everyone did not need to know all the details and responses to a person's unique questions and that the load of e-mail was becoming a bit much. They agreed that everyone wanted to be fully in tune with any health crisis that anyone experienced.

They agreed to start using closing messages on a regular basis as a way of sharing thoughts and feelings about their group process in constructive ways that addressed issues before they got out of hand. They also agreed to start using check-in messages every week, and to include in check-in personal things they wanted to share with the group. Aside from this personal sharing once a week, unless it was an emergency, they agreed to keep their messages focused on the work of the group. They agreed to respond to check-in messages one time only in the group; other exchanges about personal matters would shift to individual e-mail exchanges as often as possible. Everyone made a commitment to use their closing messages to keep in tune with how they all felt about this shift in their process.

To Deepen Your Appreciation of the Ideas in This Chapter . . .

- Think about a group meeting that you have attended recently—a group that does not yet use Peace and Power processes. Write a three-part closing that you might have shared at the end of that meeting. Consider how this process might affect the group.

- Identify a situation in your personal life that you would like to change, but that is also a safe issue to address with someone you trust. Prepare a critical reflection that addresses the situation. Let the person know you are practicing this approach, and then read or say your critical reflection. Ask the person to discuss what you have said. As an example, suppose you want to change the date for something you and your best friend want to do together. You might say: "I feel uncertain about the date we agreed to go hiking. I want to change the date to the following Saturday, because I value our time together and on that date I would not feel pressured to get back home at a certain time."

- Select an affirmation from the suggested list in this chapter. For one day, keep repeating this affirmation over and over. At the end of the day, reflect on how you felt as you repeated it throughout the day. Did you sense any difference in how you approached the day, or how you felt throughout the day?

- Continue your Peace and Power reflections for this chapter. Review your reflections from earlier chapters. Compose a closing response related to everything that you have read so far. Include a summary of what you appreciate about the book so far, your critical reflections about what you have read, and an affirmation that expresses your intention as you continue to read the remaining chapters.

Notes

1. When Charlene Eldridge and I were in the Emma Book Store Collective, the Collective used this guideline for a four-part criticism as published by Issues in Radical Therapy in 1976 in a small handbook by Gracie Lyons, *Constructive Criticism: A Handbook.* In 1988, it was republished in a revised edition by Wingbow Press. The revision remains one of the best resources for developing this important skill. The Peace and Power approach to critical reflection draws on Gracie's practical guidelines. In addition, many of her suggestions are integrated into our approaches for conflict transformation.
2. Margo Adair, *Working Inside Out: Tools for Change* (Berkeley, CA: Wingbow Press, 1984). For specific information on how to use affirmations in your personal life to create change, see Chapter 3, "Creating a Language to Speak to Your Deeper Self."
3. *Working Inside Out: Tools for Change,* p. 46.
4. Elizabeth Berrey of Cleveland, Ohio, created and owned this as her affirmation in the Friendship Collective. It is a statement that reflects what she has meant to many friends and colleagues, over and over again, in the work and play of living.
5. Notice that these questions are drawn directly from PEACE, the intent with which you enter the process. See Chapter 1.

CHAPTER 10

CONFLICT TRANSFORMATION

Conflict transformation:

- acknowledges conflict or potential for conflict early in an interaction.
- builds on the group's principles of solidarity.
- enacts the powers of diversity and solidarity.
- rotates leadership and responsibility so that those at the center of a conflict can step aside.
- addresses issues critically and constructively.
- places the conflict in a greater context so that long-term and broad-reaching implications of the conflict are clear.
- expands practices of critical reflection to embrace the perspectives of the group as a whole.
- expands practices of value-based decision-building to move beyond the conflict itself.
- brings to light what everyone can learn and how the group can grow because of the experience of transforming conflict.

Conflict is not easy, and certainly very few people welcome conflict in their lives. Conflict is often scary, difficult, painful and dangerous. But conflict is an inevitable part of human interaction, and if you want to deal with conflict in healthy and constructive ways that create safety, growth, and stronger relationships, then this chapter is for you.

Conflict transformation involves ways of knowing and doing that are central to Peace and Power processes. Conflict transformation draws especially on the powers of diversity, solidarity, and responsibility. The **Power of Diversity** means encouraging creativity, valuing alternative views, and encouraging flexibility. The **Power of Solidarity** means integrating variety within the group. The **Power of Responsibility** means owning your own actions and encouraging criticism and self-criticism in the context of love and protection for each individual and the group. (See Chapter 3.)

Even at the best of times, enacting these powers is not easy and not always possible. When a group cannot integrate diversity or variety, the group inevitably becomes engaged in divisive conflict. Typically groups deal with conflict by ignoring it, backing away from it, getting caught up in it, or agreeing to disagree. When a group is committed to the power of responsibility, conflict becomes an opportunity for growth and transformation.

To move beyond the typical patterns of dealing with conflict, it is important to realize the subtle ways in which habits of power-over powers creep into your group interactions and to develop ways to use PEACE powers. Making this shift will involve learning to embrace conflict as an opportunity for growth and an important part of group experience.

Relearning Conflict

Typical dictionary definitions of the word conflict refer to incompatibility, opposing action, antagonism, and hostility.[1] Underlying those definitions is the suggestion of the potential for violence. In fact, conflict is not always the same thing as hostility, antagonism, or incompatibility. Differences of opinion, disagreements, arguments—all forms of conflict that do not have to involve hostility or violence—happen in all groups. In a hierarchical group, a simple disagreement can quickly escalate into something that carries feelings of antagonism, polarization of viewpoints into "right and wrong," and open hostility.

There are a number of alternative approaches to dealing with conflict that are effective (conflict resolution, negotiation, arbitration, etc.), and Peace and Power approaches to conflict transformation draw on many of these. Several of these approaches focus on reducing hostilities and on an outcome of compromise between opposing groups or individuals. The best approaches seek win-win solutions.

Peace and Power is designed to move beyond these approaches in order to transform conflict itself. In conflict transformation, the group addresses the immediate issue in constructive ways but pays close attention to what everyone can learn from the situation. Everyone grows in understanding the group's values and uses the conflict process to develop new skills that contribute to the group's cohesiveness and ability to integrate diversity.

A first step in moving toward a reality where conflict is valued and valuable is to recognize the limits of adversarial definitions of conflict and to create a new way of thinking about conflict. In American English, there are no words to express the peaceful, even welcomed coexistence of differing points of view, different perspectives, or different ideas. Honest discussion can happen without hostility, antagonism, or competition for being "right." Even when people have strong feelings such as hostility or anger, transforming conflict into something beneficial for the group and for individuals is possible. Being able to do this depends on knowing that you have a choice in dealing with conflict and that you can learn ways to transform conflict.

Foundations for Transforming Conflict into Solidarity and Diversity

Conflict transformation begins before there is conflict in a group. It is very difficult—often impossible—to transform conflict by waiting until conflict happens and then beginning to work on ways to deal with it differently. Groups can develop three important traditions during times of relative calm that build a strong foundation for transforming conflict.

Nurturing a Strong Sense of Rotating Leadership within the Group

A group that has practiced rotating leadership can turn to those who have the clarity, vision, and energy to address a conflict constructively when it happens. (See Chapters 6 and 7.) Effective leadership from someone who is not directly engaged in a struggle, but who is part of the group, can refocus the group's attention. The person who steps up to provide leadership around a conflict can provide clear guidance in staying focused on the underlying issues rather than simply getting lost in the muddle of the conflict itself. Refocusing is a critical element to bring about transformation; it places the conflict in a larger context so that people can respond to the larger implications and long-term effects of the conflict.

If every individual within a group has experience at being a leader, each person already feels strong and supported in a leadership role and can comfortably move into this role when the group experiences conflict. Those at the center of the conflict can wisely step aside, hear other perspectives, and focus on their own constructive responses and actions.

Practicing Critical Reflection

Critical reflection (see Chapter 9) provides a way to learn the Power of Responsibility and to move out of communication styles of blaming, hostility, and damaging verbal assaults. Instead, members of the group develop skills of communication that focus on the group's responsibility for what happens in the group and on future possibilities for constructive growth and change. Practice in using critical reflection when no real or serious conflict is involved builds the necessary skills in a safe context and develops the group's confidence in critical reflection as a safe and welcomed process.

Critical reflection practiced regularly develops clarity about the group's principles of solidarity so that when conflict occurs this clarity is a resource for addressing the conflict. If everyone has practiced and feels familiar with critical reflection, when conflict happens and someone expands the critical reflection in addressing the conflict, it brings a sense of safety and commitment to the process, rather than the usual sense of fear and dread.

Practicing Ways to Value Diversity

If your group has established habits that draw you closer to valuing individual differences, then when you do experience conflict you will have a strong basis from which to transform the conflict. Intense feelings typically narrow or restrict your ability to remain open. Habits of valuing diversity lay a foundation to being open to many options even when feelings are running high.

The processes of check-in (see Chapter 6) and closing (see Chapter 9) are two ways for groups to habitually recognize, honor, and celebrate diversities that exist within the group. When conflict occurs, you already know and appreciate diverse perspectives, interests, and talents that individuals bring to the situation. In transforming conflict, the group's members learn more about themselves but also build on the foundation of diversity that they already appreciate.

Transforming Conflict

Whenever conflict enters the awareness of the group as a whole or of individuals within the context of the group, the group needs to address the conflict. It is always tempting to dismiss conflict as "personality differences," assuming that two or three individuals will just have to work it out. Although it is indeed desirable for individuals to resolve personal differences, conflict or hostile inter- actions within the group require a group response if it is to be trans- formative for the group.

Conflict is no one person's responsibility; no one or two indi- viduals can resolve group conflict even if they resolve a conflict between themselves. Conflict is everyone's responsibility. Every individual learns, gains new insights, and experiences new possibil- ities. As different people speak to the issue, many more possibilities emerge. The rich exchange that happens in this process brings forth many possibilities that exist among group members and provides insight from which awareness of common ground emerges.

The Peace and Power process for transforming conflict begins with someone in the group summarizing the conflict using each of the four elements of critical reflection. The process of critical reflection is then expanded as a framework for everyone to address the conflict in a constructive manner. Each person addresses each of the four elements of critical reflection, lending their individual per- spectives to the process of building a complete understanding of the group as a whole.

- "I feel. . . ." Everyone in the group addresses feelings about the conflict situation, being careful to remain focused on feel- ings without blame and without prejudging what is going on or who is doing what. It may be helpful to circle, with people briefly acknowledging their tension, anger, hurt, or indiffer- ence. Include positive feelings that can sustain the group in a constructive process, such as love, respect, hope, and trust.
- "When (or about). . . ." The group then turns the discussion to making clear what has happened to bring the conflict to center stage, acknowledging actions, words, or inactions. It is impor- tant to acknowledge individuals who are involved, without blame, but with honest and open factual accounting of agency in the situation. At this time, any misunderstandings about what has happened can be resolved, and a common ground of under- standing built.

- "I want. . . ." All members share what they hope to see happen next. Again, it may be helpful to circle so that everyone speaks, revealing as many avenues as possible.
- "Because. . . ." The group makes explicit the principles of solidarity that are emerging as central to the conflict and expresses values that are particular to the conflict itself. Everyone participates in considering how the group's principles and values are reflected in the conflict, or how the conflict can expand or change the group's principles of solidarity.

In the following sections, you will find more detailed explanation of how to constructively prepare for a discussion that involves conflict transformation. The examples show a contrast between the constructive Peace and Power processes and some of the habits that are typical in power-over contexts.

Being Specific About the Agent

One of the most familiar yet subtle power-over powers is mystification: actions that obscure responsibility for what happens (Chapter 3). Sometimes owning responsibility can be uncomfortable because you regret what you are doing or have done. Often it is difficult to own responsibility because of shyness or false modesty. Sometimes you may feel a concern (possibly misguided) about protecting someone else. Sometimes people are hesitant to name someone specifically because of fear they will offend or embarrass the person. Sometimes discomfort comes from a general sense of something that you have not thought through.

To make the shift to being specific about who or what circumstance is responsible for or contributing to a problem, consider why it is so important. Naming an instance and an agent (especially when the agent is yourself) is critical for growth to occur. If you do not know what or how to change, you cannot take positive steps to do so. When people obscure an issue or mystify a concern, others can sense that something is amiss, wonder if they are responsible or to blame, and begin to feel suspicion and divisiveness. Naming the agent helps everyone in the group to understand more about the context of the issues. It becomes possible for the group to move forward to build trust and trustworthiness because everything is in the open and everyone knows that no secrets or hidden agendas will be kept.[2]

Consider the following examples:

- *Mystifying statement.* "The checkbook ledger has been well-maintained for the past few months. This will make taxes much easier to prepare this year." Although everyone in the group may know who has been keeping the checkbook and who is going to prepare taxes, this statement discounts the individuals and makes them anonymous. It creates divisiveness because of the implied message that someone before had not done a good job of keeping the checkbook.

- *Demystifying statement.* "Anne, you have done a wonderful job of keeping the checkbook. I appreciate how much this will help me in getting the taxes prepared." This statement lets everyone in the group know how well Anne, specifically, has been doing her job of keeping the checkbook balanced. It carries the message that Anne has a skill about which others might want to know. It lets everyone know that you own the responsibility for getting taxes prepared, and that you see your task as dependent upon the work that others are doing. The focus on the present situation effectively erases the implied mystifying message about what happened in the past.
- *Mystifying statement.* "I can't stand all this clutter!" Here you are owning the fact that you see the clutter, and that you have some negative feeling about it. The mystification and divisiveness in this statement arise from the fact that each person in the group has to wonder if you are mildly irritated, annoyed, or furious. Members also have to wonder if you meant your remark for them personally or what they might have done to bring on this outburst. The matter of the clutter becomes only a vehicle for expressing your feeling, which may be due to the clutter, but it also could be directed at a person in the group whom you view as responsible for the clutter. This lack of clarity breeds distrust, suspicion, and divisive power-over relations.
- *Demystifying statement.* "I am irritated with this clutter. I am not sure who is responsible, but it is definitely worse after Jane, Randy, and Joan have been here for their publicity meeting. Maybe we need more space to store their art supplies. Or maybe we are all just getting careless about leaving things around. I am willing to help work out a solution. What do other people think?" Here you state the fact that you are not sure about who is responsible, and your uncertainty is more believable because you go on to identify a group who may be contributing more than others. You state a fact that more clutter seems to be around after the publicity group meets. Your factual statement does not in any way suggest that the publicity group is irresponsible or intentionally doing something wrong. In fact, you acknowledge that they may not have a place to put things so have no choice but to leave clutter around. You offer a possible solution and state your intention to help solve the problem.

This invites discussion and leaves you accessible to the group in the event that they find your compulsion about clutter irritating. You have left no room for suspicion, and trust and cohesiveness can build within the group because of the message that "we are in this together."

Being Specific About Your Feelings and Your Observations

A feeling statement is a precise communication of what is happening within yourself. It carries no hidden messages about what anyone else has done or is doing. An observation statement is a clear description of what you or someone else has done or said. An observation does not include what you think another person meant or what you suppose they intended.

Because owning and expressing feelings is risky, people tend to hint about something that someone else is doing or saying or use blanket labels to characterize a person or situation. Labeling a person arrogant conveys your negative regard for the person. Owning your feelings of jealousy and competitiveness because she is good at what she does makes your feelings clear without imposing a judgment on someone else. Being clear about your feelings avoids labeling, blaming, or guilt-tripping another person. It lets other people know what is going on with you in a way that invites more discussion.

Compare the following statements:

- *Interpretive/blaming statement.* "I feel rejected because I am never included in things." Even though the speaker uses the word feel, this statement avoids the real feelings of anger, annoyance, or hurt and implies what others are doing or not doing. The global phrase "I am never included . . ." invites defensiveness and resentment from others in the group. You may *think* someone has rejected you because of something that happened, but your *feeling* is anger, hurt, or fear, whatever the intention or behavior of the other person.[3]
- *Constructive statement.* "I am angry because I didn't know about the change in our meeting time." This statement expresses exactly what you are feeling, states a fact about what has happened, and can lead to a constructive response. The response might clarify a misunderstanding: "I was disappointed that you weren't at the meeting. I expected that you would be there because I left a message tucked in your door Tuesday afternoon. In the future, I will make sure that I get information to you directly."

- *Interpretive/blaming statement.* "Sue, you are so irresponsible." This statement assigns a personality trait to Sue that is derogatory and hurtful. Being labeled irresponsible invites a negative, defensive, or hostile response from Sue. Your statement is a judgment that merely intimidates Sue and everyone else in the group, creates divisiveness, and cuts off discussion.
- *Constructive statement.* "Sue, I am irritated because you have been 30 minutes late for the last four meetings. When you arrive, the group always gets distracted and we have to spend time going over things again. I am not sure how to address this, but would like for us all to discuss this issue and how we can all work together for a solution." This statement clearly expresses what you are feeling and identifies the behavior that you have observed and how it affects the group. Undoubtedly Sue will feel uncomfortable about having her lateness presented before the group for discussion. However, by inviting open discussion, you give Sue time to wait before responding and the benefit of hearing other perspectives. Group members can all enter into a problem-solving discussion without placing Sue in the spotlight or simply guilt-tripping her. In this example, everyone knows Sue is consistently late, but nobody knows why, and they have never explored the possibility that something is going on that they all need to address. Once the discussion begins with everyone willing to own part of the problem, Sue can address what circumstances in her life make her consistently late, she can participate in considering a change in the meeting time, or both. If you are tempted not to address the issue because you know Sue might be uncomfortable, consider the alternatives. Your irritation would likely grow and affect your relationship with Sue. If this is also bothering others, Sue will feel something much more uncomfortable directed toward her from the group as everyone's irritation grows.

Stating What You Want

When addressing something that needs to be done or that needs to change, provide a clear, specific statement of what you want. Focus on what you do want. Stating what you want is not a demand, nor does it mean that the group will respond by giving you what you want! It does, however, move the group toward a solution or toward a constructive response to your thoughts and feelings. If others in the group do not accept your idea, the group can sort that out and still attend to your concern as fitting for you.

Typical habits of hierarchical culture lead to two tendencies: stating what you do not want or merely implying what you want with some indirect or nonspecific comment. Compare the effectiveness of each of the following statements.

- *Constructive statement of what you want:* "I want two kids to help with this project."
- *Saying what you don't want:* "I don't think we should have too many kids on this project."
- *Implying what you want indirectly:* "Kids in this group just need to get involved."

Responding to Critical Reflection

As hard as it is to learn to be specific about who is involved or responsible in a difficult situation, it is even harder to learn constructive ways of responding when you are named as one of those who is responsible. It is much easier to become defensive or to wallow in hurt feelings. Everyone in a group that uses Peace and Power processes has to make a commitment to learning constructive ways of responding to critical reflection if everyone is to benefit from the process. Once you learn to do this, you will find that you grow by leaps and bounds, that your relationships with others will deepen and strengthen, and that your skill in dealing with difficult situations in other contexts will improve.

When you personally receive a critical reflection from someone in the group, you have at least four responsibilities:

- Listen actively, or read carefully online, to make sure you understand clearly what the other person is saying. This usually means that your first response is to paraphrase what you perceive the message to be.
- Wait for the perspectives of others in the group. Usually different people have different perceptions of a situation, and knowing these will help you decide how well the critical reflection fits.
- Weigh how fair or accurate the critical reflection is. Sometimes you will know immediately that it is fair. More often, you will need a few minutes or several days to reflect on and integrate it.
- Respond in a constructive manner. For a fair critical reflection, the most constructive response is a behavioral response: You take it to heart and change your behavior! If you decide that it is not fair, share your thoughts with the group in a constructive way.

Responding without defensiveness or apologies is difficult, and often people do not even recognize these habitual responses. Defenses or apologies do not contribute to the growth of the group, yourself, or other individuals. Compare the following responses:

- *Constructive response.* "I think that you are right, Jane. I have not realized how important this is to the group, so I will work on being here when our meetings begin." Or if you think the critical reflection has an element of unfairness: "I don't like being late either. But Jane, you have not taken into account the fact I ride the bus. I am wondering if the group could meet later so that when my bus runs late I won't be late for the meeting?"
- *Defensive response.* "I think that Jane is right, but I am working as hard as I can to be here." Or, "Give me a break. I'm doing the best I can." If you think that the group has not recognized your efforts, then share this thought with the group, but focus on what you are feeling and thinking about what you can do to address the issue of being late.
- *Apology.* "I know that Jane is right and I am very sorry. What more can I say?" You probably could say a lot more to help the group address the issue. You can also act—take steps to address the issue yourself. Being sorry does not make things right, nor does it help you or the group move forward. If you feel regret about what happened, share your feeling and suggest what you and the group can learn from the situation.

Example 10–1   Overcoming Ageism

The following situation provides an example of how a group can work with a critical reflection. This example starts with a critical reflection given at the end of a gathering, when Justa became increasingly aware of the ageist implications of a remark she made in response to Adrienne, a younger woman in the group. At the time of closing, Justa shared her criticism.

"I am uncomfortable because of the comment I made to Adrienne earlier: 'When you are older, Adrienne, you will understand.' I want to examine my own ageism because I am committed to creating a safe space here and think my remark was divisive and obstructive in contributing to that, not only for Adrienne, but for others as well."

Continued

Example 10–1 *continued*

Wisely, Adrienne did not respond immediately. Two other women in the group spoke up and tried to reassure Justa that her remark was not ageist. They thought the remark showed Justa's desire to help Adrienne. Several others in the group, however, began to share their perceptions, confirming the ageist implications of the remark.

One person said: "I felt uncomfortable when you said that, Justa, but did not really think much about it. But when you put your remark in the context of ageism, of course—it all made sense! I realize now how often I discount or overlook important signals in my own gut—I know something is not right, but I don't know exactly what. I realize tonight that I need to pay attention to this."

After thoughtful reflection and hearing others' perceptions, Adrienne could tune in to her own sense. She shared with the group that she felt angry when she heard the remark, but her awareness at the time had only been partial. Her immediate response had been to scold herself internally and to rationalize that Justa was sincere and a good person, and therefore she (Adrienne) should not have these negative feelings. She acknowledged that without the group's focus, she would have left the gathering with a sense of distance from Justa, a sense of not belonging to the group, most of whom were older than herself, and discounting her own reality. She also reflected that she probably would not have realized exactly why. Now that the group had addressed it openly, she could acknowledge what had happened. Once Adrienne focused the group's attention on her reality, everyone's awareness of ageism and its divisiveness increased immensely.

Reclaiming the Virtues of Gossip

Talk outside the group about people and events in the group, commonly known as gossip, can be a destructive source of group conflict or it can be an important source of group energy and creativity. Gossip is a skill linked with women's talk.[4] Gossip, like many other words in the English language that are often linked to women, once had a positive meaning that has now been distorted to a negative meaning. Originally, the word gossip was a noun for the woman who assisted the midwife at the time of birth. The gossip was the labor coach, and after the birth she went into the community to spread the news about the birth. She was considered a very wise woman who could communicate the wisdom of the stars.[5]

Groups can reclaim the art of gossip to develop new ways of talking about one another and events in the group.[6] The talk shared among group members in the less structured setting outside the group or in e-mail exchanges can be an important source of energy that, like the labor coach, helps to give birth to the ideas and visions of the group. Constructive and energizing gossip builds on the values of Peace and Power. The ethics of gossip that follow assure talk that is constructive and contributes to growth.

- Gossip is to be purposeful. When you tell a story about someone or something, tell why you are sharing the story. For example, if you are telling your friend about a budding sexual involvement between two members of the group, share the reason you want to talk about it. This could be because you are seeking ways to interrupt the divisiveness that could result in the group. When you and your friend both enter into gossip with this type of reason, you will move away from talk that derides, blames, or otherwise damages the people involved. Instead, your talk will focus on how the group can respond to the situation in ways that are respectful and that protect the integrity of the group. If you cannot name a reason to gossip that comes from a shared purpose, you should turn your talk to another topic.
- Own your Self. Focus on your own feelings and ideas, rather than what you think someone else felt or thought. Although you may be concerned about how other people in the group may feel or react to an emerging sexual involvement between two people in the group, focus your gossip on how you feel about it, and what your thoughts are about how it may influence the group.
- Name your source. When passing along information, be clear about how you came by the information. Share who told you about what happened, or how you know about what happened. If you cannot name your source, then do not pass along the information. Do not say, for example, "I heard that Shawna lied to her friends." Instead, say: "Jane told me that Shawna lied." Or, "I was in the group when Shawna told us what we later realized was not true."
- Be cautious about presenting information in a way that could be used to hurt another person; give information in a way that opens possibilities for greater compassion and understanding. For example, information that could be hurtful would be to

leave a class saying: "I was astonished at what Priscilla said in class today! She really is intolerant!" A message that could convey the same astonishment, but not misrepresent or label Priscilla, would be: "I was astonished when I heard Priscilla's views on the militarization of women's lives. I need to think through how to continue this discussion the next time we meet. Do you have any ideas about this?"

- Affirm the opportunity and possibility for growth and change. When talking about Priscilla's comments on militarization, examine various points that you think need to be explored to move the discussion toward constructive understanding. Gossip that focuses on what else needs to happen moves toward greater understanding of the issues.

- Use humor as a way to address emotions, and to shed light on a situation. Be very cautious about hurtful, diminishing teasing. Never knowingly tease or ridicule another person, and be cautious about humor that is self-denigrating. For example, suppose you are telling a story about being put down when you spoke up as a student in a committee meeting. A comment made in a laughing tone ("I guess I am just an unimportant student who has no business expressing my opinion") is not funny, nor is it dry humor. It is self-denigrating, and it passively implies ridicule of others about whose opinions you are only speculating. Instead, you could tell your story about how people responded to your speaking up as a student, and proclaim "Students arise!" to move toward an affirming, joyful statement that offsets your distress with the negative response you received.

- Use information to share and inform, not to manipulate. For example, if you honestly think that your friend is doing something wrong, then provide all the information you can that might help enlighten the situation without prodding or coercing your friend to decide in the direction you want. Refrain especially from making bold proclamations (which are really speculations) about the future as a way to frighten the person to decide your way. Leave the decision to your friend, even if it may turn out to be one with which you do not agree. Do not say, "You are really going to regret this a year from now." Say instead: "Let's write down all the things that might come of this one year down the road."

- Use gossip to assist and to build community, not to compete. When you hear another person's story, refrain from responding with a "one-up" story of your own. Instead, focus on sharing ideas and feelings about what her story means to you, and how together you can learn from the story. For example, if a friend tells you about a terrible thing that happened at work when they gave pay raises, do not launch into your own "ain't-it-awful" story about when your boss denied you a pay raise. Instead, say that you have had an experience that is similar, but keep the focus of the discussion on what your friend has experienced and is learning about the politics of her work life.

Anger as a Source of Strength

Anger is a feeling that many people, especially women, have learned to deny. Understandably, women have learned to fear the anger of others because it is so closely linked to life-threatening violence against women. Women's expression of anger can elicit life-threatening violence, further enforcing fear of their anger. Like the word conflict, anger is a word used in many societies to suggest many negative feelings and dynamics in human relationships.

Although anger is a fundamental feeling, other feelings and dynamics acquire the label as well. Anger is not the same thing as hatred, dislike, disgust, or envy. Emotions like hatred, disgust, or envy are not sources of strength in the way that anger can be, but these emotions need to be acknowledged and examined for their significance in pointing a way toward change and growth.

In groups committed to shifting ways of working with one another, dealing constructively with anger is a major step toward creating the safety needed to deal with conflict. Steps you can practice to learn new ways to deal with anger as a source of strength include the following:

- Recognize that your anger is a valuable tool or clue that something different needs to happen. Learn to take the time to move away from the situation until you are clear about what needs to happen differently. Use your anger as a signal that you need to step away from the situation until you think through exactly what needs to change.
- Rehearse safe ways to acknowledge your anger with people who can support your growth and understand the areas on which you are working. You can use critical reflection approaches in either role-plays you set up or in relatively safe real-life situations. Rehearse when you are not feeling angry, but work with situations that have in the past, or could in the future, make you feel very angry. Rehearsing ways to acknowledge your anger will help you overcome your fear of anger so that it no longer immobilizes you but becomes a source of strength.

- Realize that unprepared confrontation (face-to-face or online) is usually not a constructive approach to dealing with anger. Instead, confrontation usually polarizes and distances you from other people involved in the situation. Once you take the time to get clear about the signal that your anger represents, then you can think through approaches that address the situation directly and calmly, moving toward constructive changes in the situation.[7] Practice using critical reflection in groups, giving special attention to how you share what you want to happen next. Notice how the group responds to your insights and invite them to give you constructive suggestions.

Example 10–2   Writing and Power

Chullie, Justa, Lynn, Sue, and Betty formed a writers' support group and decided to meet weekly over the summer. Chullie and Justa were the most experienced writers in the group, and the other women often turned to them for guidance. One of the group's principles of solidarity, however, was to equalize the balance of power through sharing information and through valuing each person's writing skills.

Over several weeks, Justa became aware that whenever Lynn asked a question, it was directed only to Justa. When Justa spoke, Lynn paid careful attention; when others spoke, Lynn appeared uninterested. When Lynn had the chair, she looked only at Justa and always managed to sit where she could maintain eye contact with Justa. Justa became very uncomfortable with what she perceived as "shero-worship." Justa was aware that she had not yet reached full understanding of exactly what it was that bothered her so much, but she decided that she needed to address the issue in the group before her irritation became so great she could not contribute constructively. During closing at the next gathering, Justa shared her critical reflection.

> "I am growing increasingly uncomfortable—near a point of anger—every time I notice that Lynn is only directing questions to me, or mostly looks at me, and does not pay attention when other people in the group talk. I am concerned because we have made a commitment to equalize power among us, and this interaction is setting me up as an expert, at

least where Lynn is concerned. I want everyone in the group to think about this and at our next gathering share your perceptions—which may not be like mine—so that we can discuss what is going on and how we can be sure we are changing the balance of power here."

At check-in the following week, Betty responded to Justa's criticism by saying that she thought the issue between Lynn and Justa was a personality conflict and that Justa was overly sensitive about her status as a successful writer. Chullie said that she had observed—and resented—Lynn's admiration of Justa to the exclusion of others, and suggested that the group needed to look at how each person was contributing to the interactions between Justa and Lynn. Sue did not speak to the issue during check-in. Lynn began to cry and denied that she was treating Justa differently than she treated anyone else. After several exchanges that moved the group further into confusion and misunderstanding, they agreed to meet again later that week to examine this issue and to place other tasks on hold until they could resolve the conflict.

Although their principles of solidarity reflected the ideal that members of this group were seeking better ways to work together and to equalize power imbalances, they encountered a conflict that could remain isolated as an issue between two people. If they dismissed it as an issue between two people, however, the issue would continue to plague the effective working relationships within the group. By the time of the meeting to discuss the conflict, Sue moved into a leadership role and prepared a SOPHIA that consciously refocused the group's awareness on their principle of solidarity: "We will seek to equalize the balance of power among us." She placed the following subjective before the group: What are each of our perceptions of the situation now that we have thought it through? What possible new directions can we imagine to equalize our balance of power?

Chullie shared her perception that Justa often spoke eloquently to the topic of discussion, but did not facilitate other members' expressing their points of view. In fact, Chullie observed, Justa's ability to be so articulate sometimes felt very intimidating. Betty, who had not noticed any of these dynamics, shared that the open expression of the conflict had given

Continued

Example 10-2 *continued*

her the awareness that she had continued to feel like a real novice in the group and that this feeling, she now realized, was keeping her relatively unempowered as a writer. Lynn, who sincerely had not intended to treat Justa differently, began to realize that she had a habit of deferring to people she respected highly, and that her deference unconsciously sustained a power dynamic that she indeed found distasteful, but did not know how to interrupt. Additionally, she realized that she had not noticed the particular skills that Sue and Chullie also brought to the group, and had assumed that Betty was there, like herself, merely to learn how to write from the one person she saw as expert.

Once the group had entered into a full discussion of their perspectives, several things happened. Lynn consciously interrupted her doting behaviors and asked the group's feedback and support for acting on her intention to sustain mutually respectful relationships with everyone in the group.

Justa realized that she felt a certain performance anxiety to always provide answers and was relieved to be able to relax and interact without having to always be the teacher. She had not been aware that her ready answers were interfering with others' ability to contribute. She shared her intention to honor other women's contributions before assuming she had the answers. She began working with the affirmation "I value the talents of everyone in the group."

Betty gained a new appreciation for a talent she had not previously realized that she had in proofreading and accurate spelling. She made a commitment to the group to bring these skills to the group. Everyone laughed when Justa acknowledged that she (Justa) was a terrible speller and proofreader, something the group had not realized.

Sue and Chullie reflected on their experiences of taking risks and assuming the burden of voicing difficult insights about what was going on. Sue had said some brave things during her SOPHIA, and appreciated the group's responses. Chullie had confronted the effects of Justa's actions, which had been very difficult for her because she had feared that Justa might take offense. Sue and Chullie gained a new respect for their own leadership skills and ability to stay with an uncomfortable situation until it was explored thoroughly.

In this example, the key to transforming the conflict was to own the conflict as a group problem. If the group had continued to isolate the problem as existing between Justa and Lynn, nothing new could have happened; in fact, the same old patterns of hurt feelings, continued aggravation, and frustration would have persisted. In first owning and then transforming the conflict, each individual gained new insights about her unique strengths; each individual also gained self-knowledge of ways she could change and grow. This group truly moved toward honoring diversity within the group, while at the same time growing in awareness of unifying values upon which their diversity rested.

Conflict in Online Groups

Conflict in online groups can be much more challenging than face-to-face conflict; it is very easy to miss signals that conflict is brewing or to ignore conflicts altogether. Ignoring conflict might feel more comfortable at the time, but in the long run, as in face-to-face groups it festers as a negative influence on the group.

When online groups share a mutually developed commitment to address issues early and regularly practice the foundational skills for conflict transformation (rotating leadership, critical reflection, ways to value diversity), the online form of communication becomes an ideal way to address conflict. The temptation to respond offhandedly can occur online, but more often you have a few moments to reconsider and reflect on what you want to say before you hit the "send" button. You have the opportunity online to review your message, even placing it in a draft folder for a day or more so that you can gain perspective on the situation. You are able to make sure that you provide constructive criticism, that you do not imply blame or impose your own interpretations on other people's reality.

Everyone in the group needs to respond to an online message that addresses a conflict. Unlike a face-to-face group, where some members may not be present, or where some people do not speak for various reasons, in an online group, there is seldom a reason for people not to contribute to the discussion. It is wise for an online group to refrain from open discussion of the issues involved until every member of the group has sent her or his first response to the group—an online circling.

By waiting to know everyone's response, the nature of the discussion can be more focused and can take into account a complete picture of how everyone in the group feels about the conflict. If you begin open discussion before this process is complete, you can create an "e-mail hell" that results in complicating the conflict rather than transforming it.

The group may decide to call for closure of a discussion around a conflict at a specific point in time. The group may need to shift into a decision-building process to come to a mutual understanding on which they begin on a new footing. Everyone acknowledges what they have learned from the conflict, and how the group has grown in the process of transforming the conflict.

Example 10–3   Online Conflict Transformation

A class is meeting online, with the discussion focused on readings about women's health. After about two weeks of discussion, Emiko posted a message telling the group that she had an entirely different interpretation of the readings than anyone else, and that she had been offended by the Euro-centric perspective that everyone in the class had assumed was shared universally. In her message, she said:

"I am dismayed and offended that everyone's messages so far in the class have left out any responses to what I have contributed to the discussion of the readings. I have posted several messages that specifically describe my interpretation of the readings, and have explained to the group that I realize my perspective comes from my Asian and Spanish heritages. Maria, I appreciate that you acknowledged one of my messages, but not one other person in the class has responded to what I have had to say, and even more distressing to me is that everyone's messages seem to overlook the fact that there are other perspectives besides a white, middle-class point of view, even in our own class. For example, all of our discussions seem to assume that western medicine as we know it is the only viable approach to women's medical problems, without acknowledging the traditional healing

approaches that I describe as an alternative. I am bringing this to the group because we started this class agreeing that we all value different points of view and alternative approaches to women's health. I now am asking for everyone to think about our discussions so far and discuss how we can move forward in a way that acknowledges all points of view—not just mine, but everyone's. I am asking everyone to post a message in response to this message, and to not discuss it until everyone has posted."

Everyone in the group was shocked by Emiko's message. Most of the people in the group could not believe that what Emiko was saying was in fact true of their discussion so far, and went back through the archive to read the messages with this criticism in mind. Because they were meeting online, they had the advantage of being able to review exactly what had happened in the group discussion without getting caught up in "I said . . . she said" kinds of unconstructive responses. To their utter surprise, they found that what Emiko described was true; only Maria had responded once to one of Emiko's posts, and even that was a passing "thank you" and not a substantive response. More important, they realized that everyone had indeed proceeded with their discussion as if Emiko's ideas did not exist.

By the end of the week every individual had posted a response to Emiko's message. Naturally several people apologized, but focused their responses on acknowledging how easily they had all slipped into ways of thinking that perpetrated the very social dynamics that keep minority viewpoints and concerns invisible. Most of the messages shared lots of details of what they learned by thinking about Emiko's message, and thanked her for having the courage to confront the group.

They resolved over the next week to be aware not only of Emiko's points of view, but to actively seek out alternative points of view among their friends and acquaintances and bring those to the group as well. By doing this, they were not leaving Emiko with the sole responsibility of bringing alternatives to the group.

When all the messages had been posted, Emiko acknowledged that in traditional face-to-face classes she had the same experience, but had never had the courage to speak up in the past. She thanked everyone for their positive responses. After this interaction, the nature of the class discussions changed dramatically.

Interrupting Habits That Sustain Divisiveness

Divisiveness is an all-too-familiar experience within groups. Divisiveness obscures commonalities, side-tracking groups from developing solidarity in their diversity. Most of the things that sustain divisiveness in groups are habits that people have learned as the "right," "assertive," "savvy," or "political" way to deal with group interactions. In fact, these habits are rooted in power-over values, where the individual is assumed to be at odds with the group and with other individuals in the group. Integrating differences is not seen as a possibility, much less a value. This list shows examples of what happens when you are nurturing diversity, contrasted with what happens when you are engaged in divisiveness.[8]

Diversity	Divisiveness
When I am convinced that my point of view is the only reasonable one	
I still take the time to find out what other people think.	I keep repeating it to make sure that everyone hears it.
When things become tense in a discussion, and sides are being drawn	
I encourage discussion so that each point of view is presented fully.	I usually know what side I am on and grow impatient with drawn-out discussions.
In a meeting or online	
I make sure I express my point of view and limit my comments so that others may also speak to the issue.	I make sure I express my point of view at length so that others don't miss out on all the implications of my insights.
When I am aware that something I have said or done has bothered others	
I stop to consider what has happened and try to put myself in their shoes.	I figure it is their problem and it is up to them to work it out.
When others are expressing their views	
I actively listen and hear them out before framing my response. Online, I read carefully and make sure I understand their points of view.	I usually already know what they are trying to say and jump in to say what I have to say to move the discussion along.
When there is disagreement in the group	
I invite everyone to express their viewpoints so that we can all hear and consider these in reaching a decision.	I think the best way to deal with it is simply to agree to disagree and not get caught up in trivia.
When I am unable to attend a scheduled meeting or unable to be online for a period of time	
I make sure someone knows my concerns about relevant issues and is willing to take them to the group.	I figure I can catch up later and let people know what I think.

To keep sight of the extent to which your group is overcoming habits of divisiveness and moving toward valuing diversity, consider the following:

Your group values diversity and solidarity if . . .

- You can name at least one thing your group does during every meeting that reflects the valuing of each individual.
- You can identify at least two recent occasions when your group's decisions considered the minority view.
- You can identify at least three principles of solidarity held in common by each member of your group.
- You can name at least four recent occasions when the leadership in your group shifted spontaneously in response to the issue under discussion.
- You can identify (in your group's most recent meeting) at least five instances when members freely expressed appreciation for one another.
- You can describe at least two points of disagreement that your group is currently considering, and, for each of the two points, you can describe at least three distinctly different perspectives that the group is considering.

Conflict Transformation and Value-Based Decision-Building

Conflict transformation is not the same kind of challenge that a group faces when they are forming a decision, but it leads to the kinds of decisions that represent deep commitments, insights, shifts in ways of being together, and shifts in attitude. The components of value-based decision-building that are expanded in transforming conflict include the following:

- Describe the benefits that the group seeks. Many possible benefits will emerge during critical reflection, but it is helpful to be sure that the group as a whole shares a vision of the benefits that can emerge from the conflict experience. This is a key to transforming conflict, rather than simply resolving or managing conflict.
- Clarify which principles of solidarity the group seeks to bring to full expression. The conflict situation in all likelihood provides an opportunity for members of the group to grow in their understanding of what their principles of solidarity really mean when they are translated into action.

- Identify as many approaches to moving beyond the conflict as are possible within the context of the group. Transformation of conflict does not lead to one answer or solution. Rather, it leads to a number of actions, turns, or shifts in approach that are both individual and collective in nature.

When Transformation of Conflict Is Not Possible

Even when transforming conflict does not seem possible, it is well worth the effort to work toward the ideal for some time before giving up. Often, when it seems impossible, real movement toward the ideal is possible. However, when you and the group finally recognize that you cannot transform a conflict in an ideal sense, turn your energy to exploring what is possible to create better working relationships. In groups where membership is voluntary, it may be that it is time to consider ending the group altogether. (See Chapter 11.) Some voluntary groups and groups that are obliged to continue to work together might seek outside assistance in creating better working relationships. Even when less than ideal circumstances are the best that you can do, you can carry with you insights that come from the experience and build from the experience in the future.

To Deepen Your Appreciation of the Ideas in This Chapter . . .

- Think of a time that you experienced a group conflict. Identify the time when you first became aware of the conflict. Write a critical reflection that you could have shared with the group at that time of early awareness. Do you think that your critical reflection might have made a difference in the outcome of the conflict? If so, how might it have made a difference? How would you feel about sharing a critical reflection like this one in a similar situation in the future?
- Ask a close friend to role-play a couple of conflict situations with you. Take turns describing situations based on your life experiences and select the characters that you each want to play in each situation. Then improvise how the situation might unfold as you role-play transforming the conflict. Run through each situation more than once, trying on different roles and different possible responses to one another.
- Along with a friend, or in a group to which you belong, go through the list in this chapter on page 125 that helps you

identify the extent to which your group values diversity and solidarity. How many of these can your group name or identify?

🐾 Continue your Peace and Power reflections for this chapter. Think about the ways in which your understanding of earlier chapters helps you to understand and practice conflict transformation.

Notes

1. It is sometimes instructive to browse the dictionary to clarify what particular words have come to mean in popular usage, and additionally for the convoluted and interrelated shades of meanings attached to them. For instance, in *Webster's New Collegiate Dictionary,* definitions of conflict refer to "competitive or opposing action of incompatibles" and "hostile encounter." The *American Heritage Dictionary* defines conflict as "a prolonged battle; controversy; disagreement; opposition" and goes on to clarify the differences between conflict and contest. (Apparently, the degree of force involved makes a difference!) Little wonder that it is difficult to embrace conflict as a potentially growth-producing experience!

2. In an article entitled "With Gossip Aforethought" in the first issue of *Gossip: A Journal of Lesbian Feminist Ethics,* Anna Livia explains the importance of naming the agent and the source of information to build trust, especially when verbal stories we tell one another are our primary, if not only, way to find out what we need to know to work together. "It is reasonable to ask where a particular piece of gossip comes from. If a lesbian refuses to say, it is ostensibly to protect herself and her source. Why does she need protection, and from whom, if she repeats truthfully what she believes to be the truth? . . . If you won't say how you know [about a person or situation], are we to think you made it up yourself?" (p. 62). Gossip is published by Onlywomen Press, Ltd., 38 Mount Pleasant, London WC1X OAP.

3. Gracie Lyon's book, *Constructive Criticism: A Handbook,* has excellent lists of feeling words to help sort out words that carry blame from words that only own a feeling.

4. In *Man-Made Language,* Second Edition (Kitchener, Ontario: Pandora Press, 1985), Dale Spender includes a poem beginning "what men dub tattle gossip women's talk is really revolutionary activity. . . ." She goes on to note ". . . we will have to invest the language with our own authentic meanings, and repudiate many of those which are currently accented as accurate . . ." (page 5).

5. Mary Daly, in cahoots with Jane Caputi, *Webster's First Intergalactic Wickedary of the English Language* (Boston: Beacon Press, 1987). This book presents a lively discussion of gossip both as noun

and as verb in Word-Web Two. Jane Caputi, in *Gossips, Gorgons &
Crones: The Fates of the Earth* (Santa Fe: Bear & Company Publishing, 1993), expands on historical women's meanings of gossip and
shows how gossip is needed now to overcome the toxic effects of the
nuclear age.

6. Peggy L. Chinn, "Gossip: A Transformative Art for Nursing Education" in the *Journal of Nursing Education* 29:7 (September 1990),
pp. 318–321.

7. A book that I have found particularly helpful is *The Dance of Anger:
A Women's Guide to Changing the Patterns of Intimate Relationships* by Harriet Goldhor Lerner. It is a book written especially for
women who have learned to fear anger. The approaches to dealing
with anger are safe, constructive, and, most of all, achievable. She
provides useful and practical guidelines for changing interactions so
that everyone involved benefits.

8. These examples grew out of my experience with an extremely divisive work group. With Charlene's wonderful sense of humor and
assistance, I began to place myself in others' shoes to try to appreciate in neutral terms what was happening, and to understand their perspectives in a positive light. We then imagined what things might be
like in a group that valued diversity. I shared this with the group at
the beginning of a retreat, and we did experience a more positive
group interaction for that day.

CHAPTER 11

PERIOD PIECES

It helps to remember why we are doing this work. I think there is some-times the naïve assumption that if we talk about it enough, we will get it perfect, and I don't believe in perfection. I don't believe the world will ever be perfect, or that any of us will ever be perfect, or that our strategies will ever be perfect. In the effort to make social change, we learn and grow and develop, and that is what it is all about.

Charlotte Bunch[1]

Things happen in every group periodically that remind everyone of the challenges of doing the work of making change. Some of these happenings are pleasant and welcome. Others are less pleasant and unwelcome. Peace and Power processes call for an awareness and anticipation of periodic group issues and challenges. This chapter describes some things that your group can anticipate to ease the way.

Periodic Review of Principles of Solidarity

Periodically reviewing principles of solidarity is like cleaning house: It is easy to delay or neglect getting it done. Nevertheless, it is necessary for group well-being and feels good once you do it. Some groups select a season of the year as a time for assessing what is being done and thinking about changes that the group needs to make. In other groups, the time for taking a new look at the old principles comes when the focus shifts, such as when a task is completed or when group membership changes.

Three questions are helpful in taking a critical look at your principles of solidarity.

- Are we actually doing what this principle implies?
- If not, what are we doing?
- What principle is implied in what we are doing?

In the Friendship Collective, for example, we began with the principle that we would expect no financial contribution from any member in relation to our work. In practice, we encountered expenses for each person who remained a part of the group. For some women, these expenses were a problem. The review of our principles of solidarity made it possible to address these concerns and find a way to state a principle that brought the tension of unrealistic financial pressures into the open.

Open or Closed Groups?

Peace and Power groups usually seek to be open to all who wish to join. However, this is a decision that needs to be considered carefully. Some groups may not be able to be completely open because of the work they need to get done. The dilemma becomes, then, how to remain open to new thoughts, to integrating diversity within the group, and yet remain effective in your work.

One way to address this dilemma is to think of openness as relative and changing rather than as an opposing choice of open or closed. Task-oriented groups often need to maintain stability in membership to meet the pressing demands of tasks that form their central purpose for gathering. As the demands of the tasks change, a natural flow of movement occurs as some people leave the group (sometimes temporarily), and others join. Groups that are essentially permanent, such as a group that operates a community shelter, can identify times when membership is open and develop traditions to educate and orient new members.

People Joining an Ongoing Group

Integrating new members is a welcome but difficult transition. In open groups, the demands of constantly integrating new members is a challenge that requires far more time and energy than the group typically expects. Because Peace and Power groups do not function like typical groups, people who are new to the group are essentially in a foreign land, in the midst of a new culture that may be totally unfamiliar. The words spoken may be their language, but meanings of words take on a new character that existing members learn to take for granted. People unfamiliar with the language of Peace and Power often find themselves in a muddle trying to figure out what is really going on.

Once a group is committed to welcoming new members, existing members need to be constantly aware of these dynamics and establish ways to ease the transition. The group needs to set aside time to explain and clarify what is going on and to make resources such as the history, purposes, and principles of solidarity available to new members.

Groups that require relative stability in membership may set aside times during the year for orientation of new members. The group plans these events carefully. They can be face-to-face, online, or both. Members of the existing group take responsibility for various parts of the orientation. A typical new member agenda includes a history of the group, a review of the principles of solidarity, an orientation to what the group does, and a detailed description of the contributions expected of all members.

For example, in the Emma Book Store Collective, we planned new member potlucks four times a year, when those who were interested in joining the Collective could gather with us to learn about our history and our principles of solidarity and to consider what was involved in membership. We expected everyone to staff the store four hours a week and to gradually assume other tasks such as ordering new stock, managing the finances, planning for special occasions, working with other groups in the community, and taking care of the physical space. In the three months following a potluck, we expected new members to participate in each of the major activities of the business with an experienced Collective member to become oriented to the tasks. In this way, each person had the opportunity to consider making a lasting commitment carefully.

Member Leaving a Group

In groups with unrestricted openness in membership, leaving the group may be a simple matter of not continuing to contribute financially or dropping out of the gatherings or the online discussion. In groups that exist for a purpose that involves personal development, such as a reading group or a support group, the group's purpose may lead to a live-and-let-live response to someone's leaving.

However, a member's leaving the group often creates a void in the group, and people want to acknowledge the leave-taking openly in some way. In a group where an individual's leaving has consequences for other members of the group, it is especially important to state in the principles of solidarity what the group wants to happen when someone leaves. Creating traditions around this event, similar to the traditions of welcoming new members, is helpful in making this a smooth transition for the group and for the member who is leaving. Because this event represents both an ending and a new beginning, one way to approach it is similar to closing, with an entire gathering devoted to a closing concerning the leaving of the individual. Each group member takes the time to express appreciation, critical reflection, and affirmation. From this, the person leaving as well as all members of the group can carry new insights into their separate futures.

Asking a Member to Leave a Group

As difficult as it may be, sometimes the energies of the group and of an individual are not harmonious with one another. Whatever the issue is, the group must address it in some constructive way. The assumption that we can live together happily ever after is simply not consistent with reality. Ending one phase and beginning a new phase is not necessarily a failure. Still, it is very traumatic for everyone involved to acknowledge difficulty that leads to asking a member to leave.

When a group finds that an individual is not able to function effectively as a group member, the issues must first be addressed openly, bringing to the discussion the fullest of intentions to act in a way that is consistent with the group's principles. The group explores all possible avenues for resolving the issues. The discussion continues until every member is certain that the avenue chosen is one that is good for the group and loving and compassionate for the individual.

Ending a Group

Ending a group does not mean that the group has been a failure. Often it is the celebration of the completion of the purpose for which the group formed. If the purpose was not a specific task that the group can wrap up in a neat package, then knowing when the purpose has been accomplished may not be easily recognizable. For example, a group formed to provide support for one another may find that after a while, people have sources of support elsewhere that had not existed when the group was first formed. When this happens, the group may have evolved into something that is no longer meaningful. When coming to the group's gatherings or showing up online begins to be a chore rather than a pleasure, it is time to consider ending the group.

Rather than let a group simply fizzle out, plan a specific event around which the group acknowledges their ending. The event provides a means for everyone to close this phase of their experience, taking something from it into the future. Planning for a gathering for a final closing of the group online can be a rich and growth-enhancing experience.

To Deepen Your Appreciation of the Ideas in This Chapter . . .

- Think of a group to which you belong or of which you would like to be a member. Is this group open to new members, or closed? If they are open, what do they do to orient new members? Are they prepared to deal with members leaving the group?
- Consider the possibility of forming a new group around an interest of yours or a project on which you might want to work. Imagine how this group would address new members and members leaving the group. What principles would be important to you in forming this group?
- Continue your Peace and Power reflections for this chapter. What new questions does this chapter raise for you? How do your insights from previous chapters link to the questions you have for this chapter?

Note

1. From an interview with Charlotte Bunch published in *Voicing Power: Conversations with Visionary Women* (Gail Hanlon, ed., Boulder, CO: Westview Press, 1997), pp. 191–192.

CHAPTER 12

CLASSROOMS, COMMITTEES, AND INSTITUTIONAL CONSTRAINTS

Learning and teaching can take place in the interests of human liberation, even within institutions created for social control.

Kathleen Weiler[1]

The world desperately needs the new kinds of thinking that women can provide. I don't think that women are any more pure or moral than men, but since women have not been imbedded in the power structures, they may be able to provide some original thinking about strategies that are not so tied to the systems of domination. We can perhaps shake up some of the established dominations and bring in a more justice-oriented vision of public policy at a local, national, and international level.

Charlotte Bunch[2]

When you bring Peace and Power into a group that exists within hierarchical institutions, you bring a powerful influence toward transformation. You can use the methods of Peace and Power as a whole, adapt them, or use them in part for moving to new power relations in traditional groups.

The key element in making decisions about what to do and how is clarity about what value or values the group chooses to embrace. From there, the group will find many ways to enact their values. The group can then periodically examine how well they are doing in creating the value and process changes they are seeking together.

One way for groups in institutions to begin the shift is to choose one, two or three of the PEACE powers as a starting point. Many groups work within traditions that alienate and divide individuals from one another, and groups are often eager to find a different ideal toward which to work. Choosing at least one PEACE power implies a unifying value, provides a focus for the shifts in interaction, and maintains a grounding for times when the confusion of change becomes overwhelming.

The Internet and the Web, developed from philosophies of democratization, is a powerful tool for groups to use in equalizing power.[3] E-mail, distribution lists, e-mail discussion lists and bulletin boards offer equal access to information and give everyone an equal opportunity to "speak" without interruption or time constraints. As is true for face-to-face groups, everyone in the group must participate online—everyone has to show up.

People enter traditional groups such as classrooms, work teams, and committees expecting that the group will function as usual. When you present a different way of working together, explain the reasons for making the shift. If the reasons clearly relate to what the group has already been seeking, then the transition is relatively easy. The group can consider Peace and Power approaches as ways to help achieve what they already want to do.

If the group has a long tradition of working in hierarchical and power-over ways, making the transition will be more of a challenge. You might start by acknowledging a persistent problem that many people in the group see as a problem. Perhaps there is a lot of interruption and cross talk in your group discussions, and many people seldom have the opportunity to speak or be heard. You can explain your concern about this, explain why you think it would be helpful to shift to another format for discussing, and propose using a form of rotating chair to make sure that people are not interrupted when they are speaking.

Classrooms are especially steeped in traditions and constrained by institutional rules. Peace and Power approaches can be a breath of fresh air in such settings, but they can also confuse people when it is not clear why the shift is happening. The traditional teacher–student power imbalance is familiar to everyone who has attended school. The teacher has the power to grade, to offer opinions and judgments, and to speak. The institution defines the student as a receiver of grades, a receiver of the teacher's opinions and judgments, and the listener. Overcoming these expectations for roles and behaviors is not easy, and some institutional expectations cannot be ignored (such as the recording of grades to represent the achievement of a certain curricular or institutional standard).

Three values that classroom participants usually welcome are:

- empowerment for all,
- demystification of content and processes (especially processes for grades), and
- creating community.

Although you might assume that these values are central to what education is all about, they are ironically consistently undermined in most classroom situations. When a teacher brings alter-natives to the classroom that clearly enact the values of empowerment, community, and demystification, dramatic change occurs in how teaching and learning occur.

Although the values of empowerment, community, and demystification seem easy to embrace, the actual process of making the shift is a big challenge for everyone. Some people welcome the change; others respond with varying degrees of reserve, and still others object at the outset. If people who object have no alternatives, it may not be possible to make the shift. When individuals who object have a choice (for example, they can enroll in another section of a college course), they are free to leave the group and pursue an alternative. Individuals who are initially hesitant but willing to stay with the group frequently relate moving stories about the inner transformations that occur for them during the group's gatherings.[4]

Whoever introduces Peace and Power to the group may find it helpful to prepare some written or verbal orientation that is specific to the work of the group. Focus on both the value shift and the process shift that you are proposing. In classroom situations, the teacher can prepare a course syllabus in a way that makes the values explicit and reflects how the process will bring those values to life. A member of a work team can prepare a similar description for the group to consider.

The ways in which the ideas of Peace and Power influence the work of groups in hierarchical institutions will differ greatly from group to group. The value the group decides to adopt as their principle guides their choice of method. For example, if a classroom group decides to work with the Power of Sharing, there are many ways this can be done. They can share leadership through the rotating role of the convener and share participation by using the rotating chair during discussions. The group may choose a traditional lecture format for some classes as an avenue for enacting the value of sharing by the teacher to overcome knowledge imbalances. Or they can choose to have the teacher lecture for part of the class time, with rotating-chair style of discussion for another part of the time. In addition, the group can also share drafts of their written work with one another as a way to exchange ideas freely. The possibilities are unlimited.

The PEACE powers in Chapter 3 and the commitments in Chapter 4 are the basis for the suggestions in the following sections. Here the suggestions take into account typical challenges that you will encounter when you bring Peace and Power into an existing hierarchical institution. Some suggestions focus on individual behaviors, but all reflect fundamental shifts of value and attitude embraced by the whole group.

Power of Process

Required structures such as objectives, timeframes, or evaluation procedures are used as tools that provide a structure from which to work, but they are not the focal point. The process is the important dimension; the structure is only a tool and nothing more. How you interact with one another becomes the central focus. Your group takes the time to discuss your process along with the content in a classroom, or the business of the work group. Priorities related to decision-making shift, so that the urgency of making decisions lessens and the group learns to value the wisdom that comes with the process. Closing can be a powerful tool as your group learns to enact this value.

Power of Letting Go

All participants let go of old habits and ways to make room for personal and collective growth. Teachers and work-group chairs let go of power-over attitudes and ways of being; class participants and work-group members let go of tell-me-what-to-do attitudes and ways of being. Those who tend to dominate discussion let go of their tendency to speak. Those who tend to remain silent let go of their tendency to sit back and watch. All participants move into ways of being that are personally empowering and that nurture the empowerment of others. All participants share their ideas, but shift to a focus of fully hearing and understanding others' points of view.

Power of the Whole

Mutual help networks within the group are encouraged. Old competitive habits are replaced with actions that reflect cooperation. Each individual makes sure that everyone in the group has any and all information that is required to be successful. Every individual is responsible for using their talents and skills to address the interests of the group as a whole. Each participant, whether teacher or student, leader or member, is accountable to the whole group for negotiating specific agendas, keeping the group informed about absences, leaving early, arriving late, or initiating activities.

Power of Collectivity

Each participant is taken into account in the group's planning-in-process. The group works to address the needs of those who are moving into individual journeys where others may not be going. The group in some way addresses the needs of those who are having specific struggles. Individuals do not compete with one another. Instead, the group acknowledges and addresses everyone's needs as equally valuable. The group takes into account every point of view within the group in making decisions.

Power of Solidarity

The group recognizes solidarity as coming from the expression of differing points of view so that all can understand and integrate them into a richer and fuller appreciation of every individual and of the group. Out of this appreciation, each individual participates in clarifying the principle(s) that the group chooses to embrace. By actively seeking to understand the differing perspectives each person brings, the group can more fully understand what sustains them as a group.

Power of Sharing

All participants bring talents, skills, and abilities related to the work of the group and actively engage in sharing their talents. Leaders and teachers enter groups with previously developed capabilities that are shared according to the needs of the group and in consideration of the structure-as-tool. Members and participants enter the group with personal talents, backgrounds, and experiences that everyone values and shares. All participants enter the group open to what others can share and open to learning from every other member.

Power of Integration

The group acknowledges all dimensions of the situation in planning their work. Each individual's unique and self-defined needs are acknowledged and integrated into the process. Everyone—not just the leader—participates in shaping how the group's work is done. The first portion of each gathering is set aside as a time for everyone to express their priorities, needs, and wishes for the gathering so that the group can integrate these as a part of the process for that gathering.

Power of Nurturing

The group respects each participant fully and unconditionally and regards every person as necessary and integral to the experience of the group. The group plans tasks, activities, and approaches to nurture the gradual growth of new skills and abilities, assuring that every participant can be successful in reaching the goals of the group and in meeting individual needs. Critical reflection, practiced with the intention of nurturing one another's growth, becomes a powerful tool to assist one another in being successful.

Power of Distribution

Resources required for the work of the group (information, books, funds, space, transportation, equipment) are equally available and accessible to all members of the group. People share resources that individual members might purchase, such as books, equipment, or transportation (for example, through libraries, laboratories, resource rooms, or sharing among members), so that any individual who chooses not to use personal resources in this way—or who cannot—has equal access to the material. The group addresses issues arising from material inequalities among members openly to expose and overcome power imbalances perpetuated by economic privilege and disadvantage.

Power of Intuition

The process that occurs and what you address in the group depend as much on the experience of the moment as on any other factor. What emerges as important for the group to address in the moment is what happens. The group lets go of what "ought" to happen to make possible what will happen. When institutional timelines or performance expectations have to be a priority but the group also has other priorities of their own, the group weighs which priority comes first and discusses how they can still address both priorities.

Power of Consciousness

The group values ethical dimensions of the process as fundamental to the goals and purposes assigned to the group by the institution. The group considers every decision in terms of its ethical dimensions. Part of each gathering is devoted to a closing (appreciation, critical reflection, and affirmation) as a way to move to group awareness of the values represented in what is done and to consider if these are the values the group intends.

Power of Diversity

The group plans and enacts deliberate processes to integrate points of view of individuals and groups whose perspectives they do not usually address. The group deliberately includes experiences (through writings, personal encounters, poetry, song, drama, etc.) of minority groups, of different classes, of different countries, of women. Rotating chair is one way to assure that everyone hears every voice in a group, and that the diversity that exists within the group can be expressed.

Power of Responsibility

All participants assume full responsibility as the agents for their roles in the process. Rotating conveners is one way to nurture leadership. Rotating chair assures that everyone has a way to assume responsibility for what happens in group meetings. Each individual assumes responsibility to demystify the processes involved in all activities so that each member of the group has equal access to participating and understanding what is going on. In classrooms, grades become each individual's responsibility. Everyone shifts focus to what they are learning and accomplishing. The teacher or work-group leader has a special responsibility to help demystify the workings of the institution and to make explicit the political process within the institution.

Power of Creativity

The group actively seeks new and novel approaches. The group challenges and creatively reconceptualizes old problems. The group imagines and considers new solutions—including even the wildest possibilities. The group assesses that which can be retained and valued in current practices, and why. Song, dance, music, and other forms of art are integrated into the group's process as a way to inspire, to relieve stress, and to acknowledge the wholeness of experience.

Power of Trust

The group is diligent in using check-in and closing because of the value of these processes in knowing one another. Everyone speaks during these times to share personal insights and perceptions about what is happening personally and in the group. Over time, each person's integrity shines through their intentions, words, and actions, building personal knowing and trust.

Taking steps to adapt Peace and Power processes in hierarchical organizations and institutions can be risky, frightening, and discouraging. Sometimes your efforts will fail, and sometimes groups seem unable to move beyond mere token acts of working in ways that they envision. Often the hoped-for benefits and changes that happen seem completely invisible, only to become visible long after the group has ended. An important step you can take to overcome the isolation, fear, and frustration is to create a group outside the institution where you can enact Peace and Power values more fully. This is usually a voluntary group committed to working together in order to create personal and social change. Experiencing a community where you can realize Peace and Power ideals more fully, even though it may be a small group, provides a place of centering, of concentrating your energies in a healing direction, of support for the values that you are seeking to enact, and for exploring all that might be possible. Then, when the disappointments of the old world come crashing in, the visions of the new possibilities are there, somewhere.

To Deepen Your Appreciation of the Ideas in This Chapter . . .

- Think about a group you belong to that does not use Peace and Power—your family, a community group, club, committee or classroom. Select one of the PEACE powers in this chapter that you feel would benefit this group. Make a list of all the ways that your group could begin to bring this PEACE power into action. When you feel ready, share your thoughts with others in the group.
- What do you think would be the barriers to using Peace and Power in most groups you have experienced? Where you think this would be impossible, consider things that would need to shift in order to make it possible for the group to use Peace and Power.
- Conclude your Peace and Power reflections with your reflections on this chapter. As you now review your completed reflections, identify the themes and major issues that have come up for you throughout the reading of this book. What can you do to connect with others who have studied this process in order to explore your thoughts and ideas?

Notes

1. Kathleen Weiler, *Women Teaching for Change: Gender, Class & Power* (New York: Bergin & Garvey Publishers, Inc., 1988), p. 152.
2. From an interview with Charlotte Bunch published in *Voicing Power: Conversations with Visionary Women* (Gail Hanlon, ed., Boulder, CO: Westview Press, 1997), p. 188.
3. See *Democracy's Edge: Choosing to Save Our Country by Bringing Democracy to Life* by Frances Moore Lappé, *A Greater Democracy Day By Day* by Sally Mahe and Kathy Covert, and *Weaving the Web: The Original Design and Ultimate Destiny of the World Wide Web* by Tim Berners-Lee.
4. Professor Judy Lumby of Sydney, Australia, relates her experience using Peace and Power in teaching college nursing students: "We mainly used the checking in and closing processes but all were aware of why these were important. Students evaluated the course very highly. They spoke about how at first they felt that the setting and the process was foreign, but they soon felt comfortable (after about 3 weeks) and felt able to share in a way which had not been possible before. They certainly shared some wonderful stories of care from the past and present and we reflected and critiqued each other's stories to try to understand the 'why' behind our actions and how it might have been different. We found some similarities in our fears, concerns and beliefs about nursing. Students who I now meet in the ward speak about the course and say that the process was amazing for them."

BIBLIOGRAPHY

Achterberg, Jeanne (1991). *Woman as healer.* Boston: Shambhala.

Adair, Margo (1984). *Working inside out: Tools for change.* Berkeley: Wingbow Press.

Avery, Michel, Auvine, Brian, Streibel, Barbara, & Weiss, Lonnie (1981). *Building united judgment: A handbook for consensus descision making.* Madison, WI: Center for Conflict Resolution.

Baldwin, C. (1994). *Calling the circle: The first and future culture.* Newberg, OR: Swan Raven & Co.

Berners-Lee, T. (2000). *Weaving the Web: The original design and the ultimate destiny of the World Wide Web.* New York: HarperBusiness.

Bernikow, Louise (1980). *Among women.* New York: Harmony Books.

Bloom, S. L. (1997). *Creating sanctuary: Toward the evolution of sane societies.* New York: Routledge.

Boulding, Elise (1988). *Building a global civic culture: Education for an interdependent world.* New York: Teachers College Press.

Cady, Susan, Ronan, Marian, & Taussig, Hal (1986). *Sophia: The future of feminist spirituality.* San Francisco: Harper and Row.

Cameron, Anne (1981). *Daughters of copper woman.* Vancouver, BC: Press Gang Publishers.

Caputi, Jane (1993). *Gossips, gorgons & crones: The fates of the earth.* Santa Fe, NM: Bear & Company.

Daly, Mary (1978). *Gyn/ecology: The metaethics of radical feminism.* Boston: Beacon Press.

Daly, Mary (1984). *Pure lust: Elemental feminist philosophy.* Boston: Beacon Press.

Daly, Mary & Caputi, Jane (1987). *Webster's first intergalactic wickedary of the English language*. Boston: Beacon Press.

Dworkin, Andrea (1983). *Right-wing women*. New York: Perigee Books.

Edwalds, Loraine & Stocker, Midge (Eds.) (1995). *The woman-centered economy: Ideals, reality, and the space in between*. Chicago: Third Side Press.

Eisler, Riane (1987). *The chalice and the blade*. San Francisco: Harper and Row.

Elgin, Suzette Haden (1990). *Staying well with the gentle art of verbal self-defense*. Englewood, NJ: Prentice Hall.

Ferguson, Marilyn (1980). *The aquarian conspiracy: Personal and social transformation in the 1980s*. Los Angeles: J.P. Tarcher, Inc.

Forsey, Helen (1993). *Circles of strength: Community alternatives to alienation*. Philadelphia: New Society Publishers.

Frazer, Elizabeth & Lacey, Nicola (1993). *The politics of community: A feminist critique of the liberal-communitarian debate*. Toronto: The University of Toronto Press.

Freeman, S. J. M., Bourque, S. C., & Shelton, C. M. (Eds.) (2001). *Women on power: Leadership redefined*. Boston: Northeastern University Press.

Freire, Paulo (1970). *Pedagogy of the oppressed*. New York: The Seabury Press.

Frye, Marilyn (1983). *The politics of reality: Essays in feminist theory*. Freedom, CA: The Crossing Press.

Griffin, Susan (1978). *Woman and nature: The roaring inside her*. New York: Harper Colophon Books.

Hanlon, Gail (Ed.) (1997). *Voicing power: Conversations with visionary women*. Boulder, CO: Westview Press.

hooks, bell (1981). *Ain't i a woman: Black women and feminism*. Boston: South End Press.

hooks, bell (1984). *Feminist theory: From margin to center*. Boston: South End Press.

Iannello, Kathleen (1992). *Decisions without hierarchy*. New York: Routledge.

Koedt, Anne, Levine, Ellen, & Rapone, Anita (1973). *Radical feminism*. New York: Quadrangle.

Kritek, P. B. (2002). *Negotiating at an uneven table: Developing moral courage in resolving our conflicts* (2nd ed.). San Francisco: Jossey-Bass.

Lappé, Francis Moore (1990). *Diet for a small planet: Tenth anniversary edition*. New York: Ballantine Books.

Lappé, Francis Moore & Lappe, Anna (2003). *Hope's edge: The next diet for a small planet*. New York: Tarcher/Putnam.

Lappé, Francis Moore (2006). *Democracy's edge: Choosing to save our country by bringing democracy to life*. San Francisco: Jossey-Bass.

Lerner, Harriet Goldhor (1989, 2005). *The dance of anger: A woman's guide to changing the patterns of intimate relationships.* New York: Harper Perennial.

Luvmour, Sambhava & Luvmour, Josette (2007). *Everyone wins!: Cooperative games and activities.* Philadelphia: New Society Publishers.

Lyons, Gracie (1988). *Constructive criticism: A handbook.* Berkeley: Wingbow Press.

Mahe, Sally & Covert, Kathy (2004). *A greater democracy day by day.* Tulsa, Oklahoma: Council Oaks Books.

Mariechild, Diane (1981). *Motherwit: A feminist guide to psychic development.* Freedom, CA: The Crossing Press.

McAllister, Pam (Ed.) (1982). *Reweaving the web of life: Feminism and nonviolence.* Philadelphia: New Society Publishers.

Millett, Kate (1969). *Sexual politics.* New York: Avon Books.

Mohanty, C. T. (2003). *Feminism without borders: Decolonizing theory, practicing solidarity.* Durham, NC: Duke University Press.

Moraga, Cherrie & Anzaldua, Gloria (1981). *This bridge called my back: Writings by radical women of color.* Watertown, MA: Persephone Press.

Morgan, Robin (1968). *Going too far: The personal chronicle of a feminist.* New York: Vintage Books.

Morgan, Robin (1970). *Sisterhood is powerful: An anthology of writings from the women's liberation movement.* New York: Vintage Books.

Narayan, U. & Harding, S. (Eds.) (2000). *Decentering the center: Philosophy for a multicultural, postcolonial, and feminist world.* Bloomington, IN: Indiana University Press.

Noddings, Nel (1989). *Women and evil.* Berkeley, CA: University of California Press.

Peavey, Fran (1994). *By life's grace: Musings on the essence of social change.* Philadelphia: New Society Publishers.

Raymond, Janice G. (1986). *A passion for friends: Toward a philosophy of female affection.* Boston: Beacon Press.

Rich, Adrienne (1979). *On lies, secrets, and silence: Selected prose 1966–1978.* New York: Norton.

Ruddick, Sara (1995). *Maternal thinking: Toward a politics of peace.* Boston: Beacon Press.

Sandoval, C. (2000). *Methodology of the oppressed* (Vol. 18). Minneapolis: University of Minnesota Press.

Spender, Dale (1982). *Women of ideas and what men have done to them: From Aphra Behn to Adrienne Rich.* Boston: Routledge & Kegan Paul.

Spender, Dale (1985). *Man-made language.* Kitchener, Ontario: Pandora Press.

Stein, Diane (1980). *All women are healers: A comprehensive guide to natural healing*. Freedom, CA: The Crossing Press.

Walker, Barbara G. (1983). *The woman's encyclopedia of myths and secrets*. New York: Harper and Row.

Walker, Barbara G. (1985). *The crone*. San Francisco: Harper and Row.

Walker, Barbara G. (1987). *The skeptical feminist: Discovering the virgin, mother & crone*. New York: Harper and Row.

Weiler, Kathleen (1988). *Women teaching for change: Gender, class & power*. New York: Bergin & Garvey Publishers, Inc.

Wheatley, M. J. (2006). *Leadership and the new science: Discovering order in a chaotic world* (3rd ed.). San Francisco: Berrett-Koehler Publishers.

Whitney, D. & Trosten-Bloom, A. (2003). *The power of appreciative inquiry: A practical guide to positive change*. San Francisco: Berrett-Koehler Publishers.

INDEX